Infection Control in the Hospital

THIRD EDITION

AMERICAN HOSPITAL ASSOCIATION
840 NORTH LAKE SHORE DRIVE · CHICAGO, ILLINOIS 60611

Library of Congress Cataloging in Publication Data

American Hospital Association. Committee on
  Infections Within Hospitals.
  Infection control in the hospital.

  Bibliography: p
  Includes index.
  1. Hospitals—Hygiene. I. Title.
RA969.A62   1974   614.4'8   74-23438
ISBN 0-87258-148-9

AHA Catalog No. 2115

© Copyright 1974 by the
American Hospital Association
840 North Lake Shore Drive
Chicago, Illinois 60611
Previous editions copyrighted 1968 and 1970

Printed in the U.S.A.
15M-12/74-3659
6M-1/76-4914

All rights reserved. No part of this publication may be
reproduced or transmitted in any form, or by any means,
electronic or mechanical, including photocopying, recording,
or any information storage and retrieval system, without
permission in writing from the publisher.

Printed and designed by:
Visual Images Inc.
Waukegan, Illinois

Table of Contents

List of Figures vii
List of Tables ix
Foreword xi

1. Introduction 1
   Bibliography 3
2. Epidemiology of Infection 5
   Types of Infection 5
      Infections Present on Admission 5
      Infections Appearing During Hospitalization 5
      Infections Appearing After the Patient's Discharge 6
   Factors Influencing Infection 6
      Sources of Infection 6
      Microbial Agents 6
      Route of Transmission 7
      Host Susceptibility 9
      Environment 9
   Epidemiologic Principles Related to Infection Control 10
   Opportunistic Pathogens and the Compromised Host 10
   Bibliography 15
3. General Organization of Responsibility 17
   Medicolegal Responsibilities of Hospitals 17
   Infection Control Committee 19
   Surveillance and Reporting Programs 21
      Daily Work Sheet 21
      Report of Nosocomial Infection 23
   Infection Control Nurse 23
      Surveillance and Reporting 23
      Control and Prevention 26

Employee Health Service 27
    Medical Examination of Prospective Employees 27
    Treatment of Personnel 28
    Immunization of Personnel 29
    Monitoring of Personnel 31
Employee Education Programs 31
    Orientation Program 33
    Procedure Manuals 33
    Inservice Training Programs 33
    Informal Monitoring 34
Regulations for Hospital Visitors 34
    General Considerations 35
    Special Considerations 35
Bibliography 37

4. Specific Responsibilities Within Hospitals 39
    Corporate Responsibilities 39
    Individual Responsibilities 39
        The Administrator 39
        The Physician 40
        The Epidemiologist 41
        The Nurse 42
    Departmental Responsibilities 46
        The Microbiological Laboratory 46
        The Pharmacy 49
        The Central Supply Service 50
        The Food Service Department 52
        The Laundry and Linen Service 56
        The Housekeeping Department 59
        The Engineering and Maintenance Departments 63
    Bibliography 65

5. Prevention and Control of Infection 69
    Architectural Considerations 69
        Traffic Patterns 69
        Materials Handling 70
        Ventilation Systems 71
        Unidirectional (Laminar) Clean Airflow 73
        Finish Materials 74
        Carpets 75
        Handwashing Facilities 76
        General Control 76
    Environmental Control 78
        Airborne Contamination 78
        Surface Contamination 79
        Other Contamination 80
    Isolation Techniques and Procedures 80
        Routes of Spread 81
        Specific Requirements 81

      Protective Isolation 88
      Simplified Isolation Procedures 89
   Antibiotic Prophylaxis 91
   Sterilization and Disinfection 93
      Sterilization 95
      Disinfection 102
      Antisepsis 105
   Hand Washing 111
      Aids 111
      Techniques 112
   Bibliography 113

6. Special Problems 119
   Infected Personnel and Carriers 119
      Routine Search for Carriers 120
      Specific Search for Carriers 120
      Management of Personnel Carriers 123
   Hazardous Areas 124
      Blood Bank 124
      Surgical Suite 126
      Intensive Care Unit 131
      Dialysis Unit 133
      Newborn Nursery 135
   Hazardous Procedures 141
      Anesthesia 141
      Inhalation Therapy 144
      Tracheostomy 146
      Surgical Dressing 148
      Catheterization 149
   Bibliography 154

Epilog 157

Appendix A
Statement on Care of Patients with Pulmonary
Tuberculosis in General Hospitals 161

Appendix B
Statement on Microbiologic Sampling in the Hospital 167

Appendix C
Guidelines on Tuberculosis Control Programs for Hospital Employees . . 171

Appendix D
Guidelines on Hepatitis B Antigen Carriers 182

Appendix E
Nomenclature of Antigens Associated with Viral Hepatitis Type B 186

Glossary 189

Index 193

List of Figures

Figure 1
Work Sheet Listing New Nosocomial Infections 22

Figure 2
Monthly Report of Nosocomial Infections 24

Figure 3
Monthly Report of Nosocomial Pathogens and Sites 25

Figure 4
Patterns of Transmission of Infections in the Hospital 32

Figure 5
Floor Plan for Isolation Room 77

Figure 6
Card Describing Enteric Precautions 82

Figure 7
Card Describing Protective Isolation 83

Figure 8
Card Describing Respiratory Isolation 84

Figure 9
Card Describing Strict Isolation 85

Figure 10
Card Describing Wound and Skin Precautions 86

List of Tables

Table 1
Probability of Nonimmune Patients Acquiring Clinical Disease as a Result of Hospital Exposure to Infection 7

Table 2
Examples of Routes of Transmission of Infection 8

Table 3
Factors Predisposing to Infection in the Compromised Host 11

Table 4
Mechanisms by which Therapeutic Measures Predispose to Infection .. 12

Table 5
Organisms Implicated Most Frequently as Opportunists in Compromised Hosts 13

Table 6
Relationship Between Factors Causing Predisposition to Infection and Specific Microorganisms 14

Table 7
Airborne Contamination Control 78

Table 8
Evaluation of Useful Antimicrobial Chemicals 106

Table 9
Recommendations for Chemical Disinfection and Sterilization of Instruments 108

Table 10
Dressing Techniques 149

Foreword

Although there are many publications dealing with various aspects of hospital-acquired infections, the American Hospital Association's Committee on Infections Within Hospitals is not aware of an up-to-date handbook that provides in one place all the things a hospital worker must know in order to be maximally effective in the control of nosocomial infections. This publication is intended, therefore, as a handy desk reference from which the hospital worker on the job can readily obtain the information he needs.

It is the intent of the committee that the manual be an account of the practical management of infection problems within hospital units, presenting essential features as succinctly and explicitly as possible. Because there is great variation in structure, size, facilities, organization, services, and staffing of hospitals, the extent to which the recommendations in this manual can be implemented vary with each individual hospital. However, the principles presented in this work apply generally to all hospitals.

Committee members who worked on the first two editions of this manual are Maitland Baldwin, M.D.;* Philip S. Brachman, M.D.; Leighton E. Cluff, M.D.; Theodore C. Eickhoff, M.D.; Clifton K. Himmelsbach, M.D.; Robert C. Love, M.D., secretary; Joseph E. Snyder, M.D.; D. Hugh Starkey, M.D.; James G. Telfer, M.D.; and Paul F. Wehrle, M.D. The committee received able assistance from Harvey Alter, M.D., Florence M. Alexander, Louise C. Anderson, Paul R.

---
*Deceased.

Cannon, M.D., Jeanette F. Brown, Richard P. Gaulin, Clarence Hebert, Lloyd G. Herman, August F. Hoenack, Paul V. Holland, M.D., Edith A. Jones, Edwin M. Lamphere, Margaret Lamson, George F. Mallison, Bonnie B. Miller, Vinson R. Oviatt, Paul J. Schmidt, Marie M. Seedor, Milton W. Skolaut, Howard W. Spence, Wilbur R. Taylor, and Viola Mae Young.

Since the publication of the first edition in 1968 and of the second edition in 1970, advances have been made in many areas pertinent to infection control: for example, control of hepatitis and urinary tract infections, proper use of hexachlorophene, and communicability of smallpox. The International Conference on Nosocomial Infections held in Atlanta, Aug. 3-6, 1970, and jointly planned by the Center for Disease Control, the American Hospital Association, and the American Public Health Association, resulted in the exchange of much information.

The present volume is the third edition. Many sections and chapters underwent extensive revision, particularly those regarding methodology of surveillance and reporting, blood bank, surgical suite, intensive care unit, and newborn nursery. The sections on hemodialysis units, carpeting, fogging, and laminar flow are completely new. The report forms have been modified, and the appendixes have been replaced and expanded.

Committee members who worked on the third edition of this manual are Paul F. Wehrle, M.D., chairman; Philip S. Brachman, M.D.; William R. Cole, M.D.; Theodore C. Eickhoff, M.D.; F. Robert Fekety Jr., M.D.; Maxwell Finland, M.D.; Clifton K. Himmelsbach, M.D.; Joseph E. Snyder, M.D.; D. Hugh Starkey, M.D.; and Robert C. Love, M.D., secretary, who retired and was succeeded first by Bruce A. Raymond, M.D., and later by Mr. Bernard Korn. Although the text itself represents the efforts of various contributors, the committee as a whole thoroughly reviewed—and reached agreement on—all materials and issues presented.

Special acknowledgment is made for the assistance given by the Office of Architecture and Engineering, Health Care Facilities Service, U.S. Public Health Service, Department of Health, Education, and Welfare, for permission to reproduce a drawing of an isolation room; the American Public Health Association, for permission to include definitions from its publication *Control of Communicable Diseases in Man;* and George F. Mallison, chief, Microbiological Control Section, Bacterial Diseases Branch, Epidemiology Program, Center for Disease Control, Atlanta, for his cooperation in the preparation of certain sections of the text.

It was not possible to treat every facet of infection control in great detail. Some sections may be inadequate for the specialist seeking extensive advice. For those who are interested in further reading, there is a bibliography at the end of each chapter. Citations to additional references are found in the quarterly and annual editions of the *Hospital Literature Index* and in the five-year *Cumulative Index of Hospital Literature,* all published by the American Hospital Association. The section on isolation techniques and procedures in this edition has been reduced, since detailed information is available in the excellent book *Isolation Techniques for Use in Hospitals,* publication number 2054 of the U.S. Government Printing Office, Washington, D.C.

Chapter 1

Introduction

A century ago hospitals were hazardous places. Postoperative infection was so common that suppuration was referred to as "laudable pus"; its presence was thought to indicate a useful reaction to injury. Delivery of babies often resulted in puerperal sepsis and death. Very little was known about the cause or spread of infectious diseases; as a result, hospital employees, physicians, and nurses often developed communicable diseases after exposure to infected patients. Air conditioning was unknown, heating was usually inadequate or unavailable, and ventilation was provided by opening windows. Neither personal nor environmental cleanliness was considered important. Flies and other insects were regarded as nuisances rather than as threats to health. Techniques for sterilization, disinfection, and antisepsis were either unknown or unproven.

Contrast these few examples with conditions in today's hospitals. Not merely cleanliness but sterility is mandatory for certain materials. Air-conditioning and heating units with humidity control are commonplace, and air filtration is used to eliminate microorganisms. Dust is proscribed. All linen coming in contact with patients is washed thoroughly and often is sterilized. Drugs and fluids given to patients are controlled and inspected by pharmacists, manufacturers, and government agencies. Food and water are clean and generally free from potential pathogens. Patients with known infection are carefully isolated from others to prevent spread of disease. Even patients peculiarly susceptible to infection are protected against acquisition of pathogens from the environment and from other persons.

This manual is, in one sense, a testimonial to the progress that has been made in understanding and controlling hospital-acquired infections during the past several decades. Nevertheless, infections continue to develop in hospitalized patients, and may affect hospital personnel as well. Recent studies indicate that the incidence of nosocomial infections in short-term general hospitals is approximately 5 per cent. It has been variously reported that between 2 and 20 per cent of patients having surgery develop wound infection. Obstetrical, urological, neurological, and comatose patients often develop urinary tract infection. Occasional nosocomial salmonellosis still occurs. Although the incidence of infection can be reduced by increased vigilance, many other factors compound the difficulties inherent in infection control.

Human beings have always been hosts for immense numbers of microorganisms. All body surfaces harbor microorganisms; feces are composed of bacteria as well as food residue. Microbiological life abounds in man's environment. His survival in the midst of potentially disease-producing germs is due to local and systemic, natural and acquired protective mechanisms or resistances. Unfortunately, these protective mechanisms may become impaired as a result of trauma, or of disease, or of some form of medical or surgical therapy. Also, an individual's resistance to infection varies appreciably with age. As the survival rate improves, and as individuals live to older ages, the ordinarily harmless microbial reservoir in the environment is more apt to lead to infection. Thus the benefits and rewards of improved medical care and socioeconomic well-being, which permit longer life, may bring hazards.

The personal and economic impacts of infection acquired by hospitalized patients may be serious. Personal incapacitation, emotional stress, prolonged illness and hospitalization, as well as death, may be consequences of infection. Prolonged hospitalization of infected patients results in decreased availability of hospital facilities for other patients and has a significant impact upon hospital practices. The financial cost to the patient and to the hospital as a result of nosocomial infection is considerable.

In 1972, there were approximately 31 million admissions to hospitals. Approximately 5 per cent, or 1,500,000, of these patients developed nosocomial infections during their hospitalization. This represents, according to some estimates, approximately 11,500,000 additional patient days of hospitalization at a cost of $1.1 billion for direct hospital costs. Additional physician services associated with these hospital-acquired infections cost approximately $110 million. Thus, the total medical care cost associated with hospital-acquired infections in community hospitals in 1971 may be as great as $1.2 billion.

Accepting and implementing the responsibilities and measures outlined in this manual can control many infections, but it would be a mistake to believe that even their most compulsive application, or the most thorough infection control program, will eliminate all problems of infection in hospitalized patients. Further knowledge is needed of host resistance and its enhancement, of microbial survival and susceptibility, and of methods for controlling the microbial environment.

Perhaps in the future the techniques for infection control described here will seem as antiquated as the picture of hospital practices of a century ago. Thus, this manual should be regarded as advisory only. It represents what the American Hospital Association's Committee on Infections Within Hospitals considers to be the soundest information available on this subject at this time.

BIBLIOGRAPHY

American Hospital Association. *Hospital Statistics, 1972.* Chicago: AHA, 1973.

_____. *Proceedings of the International Conference on Nosocomial Infections.* Chicago: AHA, 1971.

Himmelsbach, C. K. Nosocomial infections. *Hospitals, J.A.H.A.* 44:84, Feb. 16, 1970.

Himmelsbach, C. K., and others. Conferences on nosocomial infections. *Hospitals, J.A.H.A.* 45:110, Apr. 16, 1971.

Snyder, J. E. Infection control. *Hospitals, J.A.H.A.* 44:80, June 1, 1970.

Weinzettel, R. J. Infection-control program reduces hospital stay, costs. *Hosp. Top.* 46:53, Feb. 1968.

Chapter 2

Epidemiology of Infection

This chapter presents a brief review of the types of infection, some factors influencing infection, and the types of exposure by which infection is spread. It also deals with epidemiologic principles useful in infection control.

TYPES OF INFECTION

The epidemiologic problems of nosocomial infection can be considered in three categories, according to the time of the onset of infection in relation to the patient's admission to the hospital. These categories are infections present on admission, infections appearing during hospitalization, and infections appearing after the patient's discharge.

Infections Present on Admission

Infections present on admission are clinically apparent, in the incubation stage, or in the carrier (or latent) state. In any of these situations, the microorganisms may produce illness in the patient or may be transmitted to another person within the hospital (see Appendix A, page 161).

Infections Appearing During Hospitalization

Infections that occur in patients during hospitalization, with diagnoses confirmed by clinical or laboratory evidence, are called nosocomial infections. The infective microorganisms may originate either from endogenous sources, as indigenous commensal flora carried by the patient, or from exogenous sources, as recent acquisitions from animate or inanimate objects within the hospital.

Infections Appearing after the Patient's Discharge

Some infections are incubating in patients at the time of discharge from the hospital but become clinically apparent only after discharge. Such infections not only cause an additional period of morbidity for patients, but may introduce infection into the community. Equally important, delayed recognition of the problem may permit additional spread in the hospital before corrective measures can be taken. Examples of patients with this type of infection include infants who are infected in the newborn nursery during outbreaks of staphylococcal sepsis but who do not exhibit evidence of disease before leaving the hospital; mothers with breast abscesses that appear two or three weeks after discharge from the hospital; and patients with postoperative wound infection or hepatitis B that becomes clinically apparent after discharge.

FACTORS INFLUENCING INFECTION

Many factors may influence the development of nosocomial infection. Among these are the source of infection, the microbial agent, the route of transmission, the susceptibility of the host, and the environment.

Sources of Infection

The immediate sources of infective microorganisms in the hospital are persons, fomites, food, animals, and arthropods.

Persons who may transmit pathogenic microorganisms within the hospital include all hospital personnel, visitors, and patients, whether they have a clinical disease or are symptomless carriers. Fomites, which are inanimate articles other than food, consist of medical supplies and equipment such as furniture, blankets, humidifiers, anesthesiology equipment, drugs, and solutions. Such solutions may include intravenous solutions contaminated by bacteria or fungi or blood or its products contaminated by hepatitis virus. Occasionally, food and water contaminated by salmonella or shigella microorganisms have been sources of nosocomial infection. In some instances animals or insects are important sources.

Microbial Agents

There are many kinds of pathogens to which a patient may be exposed during hospitalization. The likelihood of infection resulting from such exposure depends in part on the species of pathogen, its resistance to antimicrobial agents being administered to the patient, its virulence, and the numbers introduced to the patient (see Table 1, opposite). Depending on the method of transmission and host factors, any microorganism can be a pathogen.

Table 1
PROBABILITY OF NONIMMUNE PATIENTS ACQUIRING CLINICAL DISEASE AS A RESULT OF HOSPITAL EXPOSURE TO INFECTION

Probability	Disease
High (50% or more)	Chickenpox Influenza Measles (rubeola) Mumps Plague, pneumonic Rubella (German measles) Smallpox Whooping cough (pertussis)
Medium (10 to 50%)	Acute viral respiratory disease (common cold) Hepatitis A (infectious hepatitis) Hepatitis B (serum hepatitis) Shigellosis Streptococcal infections
Low (less than 10%)	Amebiasis Diphtheria Meningococcal infections Poliomyelitis and other enterovirus infections Salmonellosis-typhoid Staphylococcal infections Tuberculosis

Route of Transmission

As noted in Table 2, next page, microorganisms can be transmitted within the hospital environment by any of four routes: contact, air, a common vehicle, or a vector. More than one route may be operational in the transmission of a pathogen during a single episode, and the same pathogen can be transmitted by different routes on different occasions.

Contact transmission can occur by the direct, indirect, or droplet route. *Direct* contact transmission refers to spread from the source to a recipient directly without an intermediary object—for example, the fecal-oral spread of hepatitis via contaminated hands. Staphylococci can also be transmitted by the direct contact route. *Indirect* spread indicates that the organisms are transferred from the source to a recipient via an intermediary object—for example, gram-negative septicemia resulting from infusion of contaminated intravenous fluids. *Droplet*-spread diseases are those whose infectious agents are transmitted from the source in the form

Table 2
EXAMPLES OF ROUTES OF TRANSMISSION OF INFECTION

Mode	Type	Disease
Contact	Direct	Hepatitis A Gonorrhea Syphilis Staphylococcal infections (some)
	Indirect	Pseudomonas infections (some) Malaria (needle) Hepatitis B
	Droplet	Measles Streptococcal pharyngitis
Airborne	Droplet nuclei	Chickenpox Tuberculosis Diphtheria
	Dust	Tetanus Gas gangrene
Common vehicle	Foodborne	Salmonellosis Staphylococcal gastroenteritis
	Waterborne	Shigellosis Cholera
Vectorborne	Mosquito	Malaria
	Flea	Bubonic plague
	Tick, mite, louse	Rickettsial diseases

Many of these diseases may be transmitted by more than one route.

of droplets to a recipient who is within several feet of the source—for example, streptococcal disease and influenza. Droplets never become independently airborne.

Airborne organisms are spread either in droplet nuclei or resuspended dust. Droplet nuclei are particles whose physical characteristics permit them to be transmitted more than several feet and remain suspended in the air for long periods of time. Diseases that may be spread by airborne droplet nuclei are tuberculosis, smallpox, and varicella.

Common vehicle means that multiple cases of a disease are related to the same source of infection; food or water usually serves as the common vehicle. Such diseases as salmonellosis and staphylococcal gastroenteritis are often foodborne; shigellosis can be spread by the waterborne route.

Vectorborne diseases, such as malaria, are no longer common in the United States.

Some etiologic agents can be transmitted by more than one route. For example, staphylococci can be transmitted by contact, air, or a common vehicle, though the most common route is direct contact.

Host Susceptibility

Significant factors in the host include age, immune status, type of underlying disease, and effects of diagnostic and therapeutic procedures. For example, the extremes of life—infancy and old age—are associated with a decreased resistance to infection. Patients with chronic disease, such as certain types of cancer, leukemia, diabetes mellitus, lymphoma, or nephrosis, may be more susceptible to nosocomial infection than other patients. Additional host factors are nutritional status, alcoholism, lowered local resistance, and hypogammaglobulinemia.

Many diagnostic procedures, such as biopsy, catheterization, and aspiration of fluid, tend to increase the patient's risk of infection. Some therapeutic procedures, such as surgery, use of antibiotics, ionizing radiation, and treatment with immunosuppressive drugs, also are associated with increased susceptibility to infection.

Environment

A wide variety of pathogenic organisms is introduced into the hospital environment. Through selection, the use of antibiotics has led to the emergence of drug-resistant strains of bacteria. Such bacteria may become more difficult to manage than nonhospital-related strains. This difficulty may become especially evident in hospital areas such as surgical services, where approximately one-half of all nosocomial infections occur.

Microorganisms shed from infected lesions may also be more virulent than those ordinarily found in the inanimate environment. Patients infected at the time of admission may carry especially virulent strains of microorganisms, which later may tend to predominate in the hospital environment.

Selection of antibiotic-resistant strains involves more than a single mechanism. With the staphylococci, for example, the operative mechanism may be simply that of selection of resistant variants, whereas among enteric bacteria there may also be transfers of resistance factors (R).

Crowded conditions within the hospital also favor transmission of microorganisms. In addition, changes in temperature or humidity may at times influence the development of infection. Moreover, the development of the carrier state in hospital personnel or patients may lead to difficult problems of control, as was clearly evident in an interstate epidemic of *Salmonella derby* infection involving many hospitals.

EPIDEMIOLOGIC PRINCIPLES RELATED TO INFECTION CONTROL

Certain information is helpful in ascertaining the presence of an outbreak of infection in a hospital and subsequently in breaking the chain of transmission of infective microorganisms. The answers to these questions should help an infection control committee determine whether or not the hospital is experiencing a problem in infection control.

- Are the data on frequency of infection on a particular service or on all services comparable to previous data on the same services in the same hospital? The data should be analyzed for overall disease incidence as well as for specific diseases. It may be possible to compare these data to similar data from other hospitals, but this must be done with great care, since there are potentially great differences in the incidence of infection among hospitals that handle different types of patients and perform different procedures.
- Are there trends of disease on one or more services that suggest that a problem may exist? Because most outbreaks of nosocomial disease exhibit an increased incidence over a period of days or weeks before an epidemic is recognized, surveillance information should be gathered and analyzed at regular intervals.
- Is the type of clinical infection under scrutiny unusual for the particular hospital?
- Have uncommon microorganisms been identified? For example, detection of only a few salmonella infections of unusual type may warrant detailed investigation, or an increase in a common microorganism such as *Staphylococcus aureus* might indicate an epidemic.
- Are the infected patients under review unusual in relation to age, underlying disease, sex, or domiciliary location; and do their infections reflect an unusual number of admissions with unexpected underlying problems?
- Is there a possibility of a common source of infection? Have the patients had similar procedures, the same physician or surgeon, identical special services, or other common hospital experiences?
- In the judgment of the infection control committee, are special investigative or control measures indicated?

OPPORTUNISTIC PATHOGENS AND THE COMPROMISED HOST

Microorganisms capable of causing infectious disease in healthy persons are commonly referred to as pathogens. Less pathogenic micro-

Table 3
FACTORS PREDISPOSING TO INFECTION IN THE COMPROMISED HOST

Group	Factor

Circumvents external anatomical barriers	Burns, extensive dermatitis
	Catheters, intravenous and urinary
	Decubiti
	Impairment of the tracheobronchial mucociliary escalator
	    Cold
	    Smoke
	    Drugs (alcohol, anesthetics)
	Influenza (necrotizing tracheitis)
	Injections, diagnostic procedures
	Neurological disorders altering consciousness
	Surgery
	Trauma

Impairs granulocyte behavior and cellular immunity	Adrenal steroid therapy Alcoholism Antineoplastic drugs Anergic states, as in sarcoidosis Burns Collagen-vascular diseases Complement (C3 and C5) deficiencies (chemotaxis deficiencies) Congenital defects of cellular immunity Congenital disorders of leukocyte or lysosomal function Congestive heart failure Diabetes mellitus, especially with acidosis Foreign bodies (valves, grafts, shunts, catheters) Hemoglobinopathies Immunologic deficiency syndromes Immunosuppressive drugs Ionizing radiation Leukemia Lymphoma, Hodgkin's disease, myeloma Malignancies, especially gastrointestinal or advanced Malnutrition Neutropenia (granulocytopenia $< 1,000/mm.^3$) Obstruction of bronchi, biliary tract, ureter Old age Organ transplants (renal) with use of immunosuppressive techniques Shock Splenectomy Surgical creation of dead spaces, hemotomas, tissue necrosis Uremia, especially with acidosis Vascular insufficiency, gangrene
Impairs immunoglobulin defenses	Cirrhosis Complement defects Congenital and acquired immunoglobulin deficiencies Dysproteinemias Splenectomy

Affects microbial load or dose	Antimicrobial drug-induced alterations in flora
	Changes in normal flora with serious disease per se
	Disseminating carriers
	Environmental reservoirs
	    Contaminated equipment
	    Contaminated medications
	Food and water
	Improper isolation procedures
	Nursing and housekeeping practices

organisms are capable of causing disease in persons whose defense mechanisms are deficient or compromised; therefore, these microorganisms are often referred to as opportunistic pathogens. Commensals that normally inhabit skin, mucous membranes, and the gastrointestinal tract are frequent opportunists. Saprophytes that exist abundantly in our environment, where they are ordinarily of little concern, also may invade weakened patients. Some of the important factors that impair host defenses and predispose persons to opportunistic pathogens are summarized in Table 3, previous page.

Persons with deficient defense mechanisms are found most frequently in hospitals. Thus, infections caused by opportunistic pathogens may be expected most frequently among hospitalized patients. These infections arise with increasing frequency as noncurative therapeutic measures become more and more effective in prolonging the lives of seriously ill

Table 4

MECHANISMS BY WHICH THERAPEUTIC MEASURES PREDISPOSE TO INFECTION

Therapy	Effect
Antimicrobial drugs	Alter normal flora and select resistant types May encourage growth of some fungi May alter immunoglobulins in sera
Corticosteroids	Depress antibody formation Depress reticuloendothelial cellular function Promote the diabetic state Suppress granulocyte responses Suppress interferon production Suppress lymphocytes and mononuclear cells needed for cellular immunity reactions
Ionizing radiation	Depresses antibody formation Depresses bone marrow production of leukocytes Depresses granulocyte function Injures tissues, producing portals of entry and other structural derangements hindering drainage and defense mechanisms Suppresses the reticuloendothelial system
Antimetabolites and antineoplastic drugs	Produce changes similar to ionizing radiation above
Surgical procedures and insertion of foreign material	Provide portal of entry to highly susceptible tissues Provide a mechanism for persistence of organisms

patients. Opportunistic infections often occur following successful antibiotic treatment of serious infections caused by virulent pathogens. The weakened patient is then victimized by less pathogenic organisms from his environment (exogenous infection) or from his own flora (endogenous infection). Secondary infections are particularly difficult to treat, and their victims have a high mortality rate even though the infections may be caused by relatively less virulent bacteria.

Antibiotics are by no means the only therapeutic measures that have been implicated in the development of opportunistic infections. Medications widely used in the treatment of malignancies and various chronic diseases may delay or diminish the leukocytic inflammatory reaction that is helpful in containing microorganisms. Cellular immune deficiencies are associated with severe bacterial, fungal, viral, and parasitic infections. Therapeutic measures that predispose persons to opportunistic infection are listed in Table 4, opposite.

Practically any organism can infect weakened and debilitated patients. The isolation of an organism from some site in or on the body does not

Table 5
ORGANISMS IMPLICATED MOST FREQUENTLY AS OPPORTUNISTS IN COMPROMISED HOSTS

Group	Organism
Bacteria	Bacteroides
	Escherichia coli
	Enterobacter species
	Enterococci
	Flavobacteria
	Klebsiella pneumoniae
	Mycobacteria
	Nocardia asteroides
	Proteus species
	Providencia
	Pseudomonas aeruginosa
	Serratia marcescens
	Staphylococcus aureus
	Staphylococcus epidermidis (albus)
Fungi	Aspergillus
	Candida
	Cryptococcus
	Histoplasma
	Phycomycetes (Mucor)
Viruses	Cytomegalovirus
	Hepatitis B
	Herpesvirus hominis 1 and 2
	Vaccinia
	Varicella-zoster
Parasites	*Pneumocystis carinii*
	Strongyloides stercoralis
	Toxoplasma gondii

always mean the organism is causing a disease requiring antibiotic therapy. The most troublesome organisms are listed in Table 5, previous page, and some of the associations between specific disease states and various organisms are shown in Table 6, below.

Table 6

RELATIONSHIP BETWEEN FACTORS CAUSING PREDISPOSITION TO INFECTION AND SPECIFIC MICROORGANISMS

Factor	Organism
Extensive abdominal surgery	Gram-negative bacilli Bacteroides and anaerobic streptococci Staphylococci
Burns, trauma	Pseudomonas, Serratia, Proteus, staphylococci, Candida, Mucor
Cardiac surgery	Staphylococci *(aureus, epidermidis)* Gram-negative bacilli Candida Diphtheroids
Intravenous catheters	Staphylococci Pseudomonas Candida Mimae
Urinary tract instrumentation	Gram-negative bacilli Enterococci
Tracheostomy, nebulizers, respirators	Pseudomonas, Klebsiella Serratia Staphylococci Candida
Agranulocytosis	Pseudomonas Staphylococci
Diabetes mellitus	Staphylococci Mucor, Candida Gram-negative bacilli
Immunosuppressive or antimetabolite therapy for neoplasms, leukemia, lymphomas, connective tissue diseases, and renal or cardiac transplant	Pseudomonas Klebsiella, Enterobacter, Serratia Staphylococci Diphtheroids Listeria Nocardia Candida Aspergillus Cryptococcus Cyptomegalovirus Herpes zoster *Pneumocystis carinii* Phycomycetes

Some of the factors predisposing hosts to opportunistic infections do so by facilitating the entry of microorganisms into tissues, thus enabling them to circumvent the body's natural defenses. Surgical procedures are the outstanding example. Indwelling urinary and intravenous catheters are also important examples, especially because they are commonplace and often avoidable. Anesthetics and other drugs have been incriminated in the development of pneumonia in hospitals, because their altering of the sensorium may result in the aspiration of pharyngeal secretions and organisms. Ultrasonic nebulizers and equipment used for inhalation therapy may become heavily colonized with opportunistic organisms, particularly pseudomonas and serratia, and may be responsible for nosocomial epidemics of pneumonia. These and a few other organisms are noteworthy for their ability to survive and even multiply in aqueous solutions and medications that nonetheless may remain clear and seemingly safe for patients use.

Antimicrobial drugs given prophylactically are not a satisfactory long-term solution to the problem of opportunistic pathogens, because of the changing selection of organisms resistant to the antibiotics in use. Organisms will always be available to cause disease in highly susceptible hosts.

Opportunistic infections in compromised hosts, although seemingly inevitable, can be reduced by:

- Appreciation of the importance of preserving normal defenses, and elimination, whenever possible, of all factors that compromise the host.
- Efforts (such as reverse isolation) to minimize the exposure of susceptible tissues to dangerous organisms.
- Early diagnosis and optimal treatment of opportunistic infections.

BIBLIOGRAPHY

FACTORS INFLUENCING INFECTION

Datta, N. Infectious drug resistance. *Brit. Med. Bull.* 21:254, Sept. 1965.

Elek, S. D. *Staphylococcus Pyogenes and Its Relation to Disease.* Baltimore: Williams & Wilkins, 1959.

―――――――. Experimental staphylococcal infections in the skin of man. *Ann. N.Y. Acad. Sci.* 65:85, Aug. 31, 1956.

Mailbach, H. A., and Hildrick-Smith, G., editors. *Skin Bacteria and Their Role in Infection.* New York: McGraw-Hill, 1965.

Sanders, E., and others. An outbreak of hospital-associated infections due to *Salmonella derby. J. Amer. Med. Assn.* 186:984, Dec. 14, 1963.

Watanabe, T. Infective heredity of multiple drug resistance in bacteria. *Bact. Rev.* 27:87, Mar. 1963.

EPIDEMIOLOGIC PRINCIPLES

American Public Health Association. *Control of Communicable Diseases in Man.* 11th ed. New York: APHA, 1970.

Streeter, S., and others. Hospital infection—a necessary risk? *Amer. J. Nurs.* 67:526, Mar. 1967.

Williams, R. E. O., and others. *Hospital Infection: Causes and Prevention.* 2nd ed. Chicago: Year Book Publishers, Inc., 1966.

Williams, R. E. O., and Shooter, R. A., editors. *Infection in Hospitals: Epidemiology and Control.* A symposium organized by the Council for International Organizations of Medical Sciences, under the joint auspices of UNESCO and WHO. Philadelphia: F. A. Davis Co., 1963.

OPPORTUNISTIC PATHOGENS AND THE COMPROMISED HOST

Burke, J. F. Clinical determinants of host susceptibility to infection in surgical patients. In: *Proceedings of the International Conference on Nosocomial Infections.* Chicago: American Hospital Association, 1971, pp. 169-72.

Cluff, L. E. Medical determinants of nosocomial infections. In: *Proceedings of the International Conference on Nosocomial Infections.* Chicago: American Hospital Association, 1971, pp. 164-68.

Fekety, F. R., Jr., and Murphy, J. F. Factors responsible for the development of infections in hospitalized patients. *Surg. Clin. N. Amer.* 52:1385, Dec. 1972.

Klainer, A. S., and Beisel, W. R. Opportunistic infection: a review. *Amer. J. Med. Sci.* 258:431, Dec. 1969.

GENERAL READINGS

American Hospital Association. *Proceedings of the International Conference on Nosocomial Infections.* Chicago: AHA, 1971.

National Library of Medicine. *Literature Search 32-65; Hospital-Acquired Infections, Jan. 1964-Oct. 1965 (276 citations).* Bethesda, Md.: NLM, 1965.

Chapter 3

General Organization of Responsibility

This chapter contains guidelines for establishing an infection control committee. It also suggests programs, services, and regulations of a general nature to help the infection control committee in its work to control and prevent nosocomial infections.

MEDICOLEGAL RESPONSIBILITIES OF HOSPITALS

It is assumed that interest in patient care will cause most hospitals to undertake to comply with standards for infection control that have been adopted under various state licensing regulations and the Joint Commission on Accreditation of Hospitals (JCAH). There may also be considerations of legal liability that support this natural interest.

If a patient can establish that he incurred an infection and thereby suffered injury as a result of the negligence of a hospital or its employees, or as a result of the hospital knowingly permitting members of its medical staff to employ nonaseptic techniques, the institution itself may be legally liable for those injuries. Important as this consideration is, it should nevertheless be secondary to the primary interest in patient care.

In determining the standards of care within a hospital, the courts of some states restrict a comparison to other hospitals in the same or like communities. In other states, the comparison may be to the industry as a whole. No matter which standard is found applicable by a state's courts, there will nevertheless be an opportunity for the injured plaintiff to show, if he can, that the hospital standard of care did not conform to that standard.

Applicable standards can certainly be found within the hospital's own written policies. In most states, certain of these standards can be found within the state hospital licensing regulations. In a hospital accredited by the JCAH, standards can also be found for legal purposes within the JCAH's standards. In the famous Darling case,* the Illinois Supreme Court held that general custom by hospitals is also relevant in determining a legal standard of care and that hospital licensing standards, accreditation standards, and a hospital's bylaws could be persuasive to the jury, if not legally conclusive, as to what an applicable standard may be. Although not necessarily reaching the same ultimate conclusion as the Illinois case, the courts of other states have reached a similar conclusion as to the relevance and persuasiveness of such documents.

It is to be remembered, of course, that compliance with standards of this type does not necessarily ensure that a defendant will be exonerated from liability. It is recognized that prevailing standards of an industry may be inappropriate to establish a legally acceptable standard of care, in which case compliance with such standards will not assist the defendant.

On the other hand, there are those who are tempted to believe that adoption or compliance with standards is inherently dangerous at law and should be avoided. Courts have countered this philosophy in some states by holding that the failure to adopt a standard can also be proof of negligence and can therefore incur liability.

In the interest of patient care and with a prudent eye on potential liability, hospitals would do well to consider the adoption of the minimal standards of infection control that have been recommended by the American Hospital Association and the JCAH. Although accreditation standards may pertain directly only to accredited hospitals, a sufficient number of hospitals within the comparison area may be accredited or may subscribe to accreditation standards so as to make those accreditation standards the prevailing standard of the area. Thus, a nonaccredited hospital may be held to the standards of accreditation.

Standards established by the JCAH require hospitals to provide at least:
- An infection control committee that maintains surveillance services.
- A sanitary environment.
- Facilities for the isolation of infected patients.
- A competent and adequate microbiology service.
- Restricted duties for obstetrical nurses.
- Adequate protection against contamination of foods.

Darling v. Charleston Community Memorial Hospital, 211 N.E. 2d 253 (Ill. 1965), *cert. denied* 383 U.S. 946 (1966).

It should follow as a matter of course that hospitals would comply with all applicable licensing regulations on the subject. Because both failure to comply with standards and even failure to adopt standards can be equally dangerous at law, humanitarian considerations should prompt compliance with applicable standards and adoption of such standards where they do not exist.

INFECTION CONTROL COMMITTEE

The reponsibility of the hospital for the prevention and control of infection extends to its patients and personnel, and to those who are visiting patients. In order to provide guidelines for hospitals in the fulfillment of these responsibilities, the Committee on Infections Within Hospitals of the American Hospital Association developed and published (as an article in *Hospitals, J.A.H.A.*) recommendations in 1958, and later expanded them in the 1968 and 1970 editions of the present manual.

Consistent with its previous recommendations and those of the JCAH, the AHA's current recommendations for the hospital's role in infection control are:

1. Each hospital shall establish a committee on infection control.
2. This committee shall meet regularly and upon special indication.
3. Membership on this committee should include representation of the following: hospital administration, internal medicine, microbiology (pathology), nursing, obstetrics, pediatrics, and surgery. In addition, consideration should be given to regular or ad hoc participation by representatives of other departments, including blood bank, dietetics, employee health, housekeeping, house staff, outpatient, and pharmacy.
4. The committee shall be responsible for the following functions:
   - Establish and operate a practical system for reporting and evaluation of infections in patients, personnel, and discharged patients.
   - Distinguish between nosocomial infections and those not causally associated with hospitalization.
   - Attempt to identify the source and method of transmission of each nosocomial infection.
   - Make recommendations and take appropriate measures to limit further spread from identified sources of contagion.
5. In order to be maximally effective in controlling nosocomial infections, the committee should:
   - Make certain that reliable microbiological services are available.

- Be provided with the assistance of an infection control nurse and/or an epidemiologist. Consideration should be given to designating a qualified committee member to serve as the hospital epidemiologist or infection control officer. The infection control officer, assisted by an infection control nurse, supervises the infection surveillance program, determines sources of infection, consults on isolation and control of infectious diseases, serves as liaison with the health department, plans orientation and training programs, and so forth.
- Make definitive provision for adequate isolation policies and procedures.
- Make certain that all personnel are instructed in the proper practice of medical and surgical asepsis and in their respective roles and responsibilities in the prevention and control of nosocomial infections.
- Regularly analyze data on infections, evaluate current trends and experience, and undertake such control measures as may be indicated.
- Regularly prepare and distribute to the hospital staff those reports that are pertinent to infection control.
- Provide counsel and advice on infection control.
- Review practices and procedures that tend to compromise patients' resistance to infection, such as chemoprophylaxis; immunosuppression by drugs; instrumentation, intubation, and catheterization; and ionizing radiation.
- Conduct prevalence studies to spot-check on the adequacy of reporting.
- Monitor antibiotic usage.
- Review and update the control program periodically.
- Coordinate infection control practices with those of other hospitals in the community in order to facilitate consistent implementation of these practices by physicians and allied health personnel who serve in more than one hospital.
- Coordinate procedures for isolation of patients.
- Report specific notifiable infections to the health authorities.
- Maintain continuing communication and close cooperation with the appropriate committee of the local medical society, in order to exchange information on infections and to facilitate the follow-up of patients discharged from the hospital.

SURVEILLANCE AND REPORTING PROGRAMS

The purpose of an infection surveillance program is to detect and record nosocomial infection in a systematic fashion in order to institute the most effective and practical control procedures. Knowledge of the usual endemic rate of infection in a hospital enables infection control personnel to detect potential epidemics and to identify areas in need of investigation or more specific control measures. Such information can also be useful in teaching programs within the hospital and in evaluating the effectiveness of new control measures.

Experience has shown that no single surveillance system will provide complete information on the frequency of nosocomial infection (see Appendix B, page 167). Therefore, a combination of several techniques, suitable to the hospital's program, is recommended. Among these are:
- Daily review of all culture requests and reports in the microbiology laboratory. All reports suggestive of hospital infections must be followed up by reviewing the clinical records on the wards.
- Frequent, daily if possible, chart checks on each nursing unit for clues to the possible presence of infection (fever, isolation, soaks, antibiotic use, doctors' or nurses' notes).
- Reports in an infection log kept on each nursing unit.
- Reports by physicians or charge nurses.
- Prevalence surveys conducted at regular intervals (such as quarterly) in order to validate the surveillance data, permit an evaluation of antibiotic usage, and serve as an educational benefit to the hospital staff.

In any event, regular input of hospitalwide information on the occurrence of infection is vital to the success of an infection control program. How best to accomplish this depends on the characteristics of the individual hospital.

The following suggestions describe a useful set of procedures that can be easily adapted to the needs of most hospitals. Surveillance can be accomplished with the use of three basic reporting forms: a daily work sheet (Figure 1, next page), and two monthly summary forms (Figures 2 and 3, pages 24 and 25). Other forms can be developed as required, such as those noting infections present on admission.

Daily Work Sheet

A daily work sheet form (Figure 1, next page) is used by the infection control nurse to maintain a continuing record of each infection. The amount of information recorded will depend on the person recording it—

Patient's last name, first initial	Patient's hospital number	Physician's name	Date of admission	Date of onset	Age	Sex	Service	Ward	Site infected	Antibiotics used	Pathogen(s) antibiogram	Type of treatment or procedure, and date	Underlying problem

Figure 1

WORK SHEET LISTING NEW NOSOCOMIAL INFECTIONS

the nurse, hospital epidemiologist, infection control committee—and on what use will be made of the data. The category "host factors" can include diseases or procedures that may increase host susceptibility to infection, such as malignancy, radiation therapy, or urinary catheters. This record should be reviewed weekly with the hospital epidemiologist to check for evidence of clusters of infections.

Report of Nosocomial Infection

The monthly statistical summaries (Figures 2 and 3, next two pages) are prepared by the infection control nurse. Using the hospital discharge statistics by service and the individual patient infection reports, the nurse can calculate the rates of nosocomial infections for the entire hospital, for major services, and by types of infection. These data should be reviewed monthly by the infection control committee. The committee also should make the data available to staff members on a regular basis, since effective surveillance consists not only of the collection of information but also of its synthesis and interpretation for those who contributed to it.

As special problems develop, other summary forms should be prepared. For example, a service-pathogen grid chart would be very useful in making analyses when an increased frequency of a pathogen on a particular service is noted.

Individual patient reporting forms have been used in some institutions, but they have not proven to be effective and are not recommended.

INFECTION CONTROL NURSE

The surveillance activities of the infection control nurse will differ in each hospital, depending on the hospital's characteristics and surveillance program. Another variable will be the time the nurse has available for this function. Accordingly, some or all of the following duties may be included in the job description:

Surveillance and Reporting

- Make regular ward rounds seeking clues of infection (fever, isolation, soaks, use of antibiotics); discuss possible infections with charge nurse. The frequency of reviews would vary from daily to weekly, depending upon the frequency of infections, type of hospital, and available time.
- Check daily with the microbiological laboratory for the presence of cultures that might represent developing infection, and follow up as indicated.

Number of patients with one nosocomial infection _____
Number of patients with two nosocomial infections _____
Number of patients with three or more nosocomial infections _____
                                                 Total _____

Month/year

	Number	% of discharges
	_____	_____
	_____	_____
	_____	_____
Total	_____	100%

Number of hospital discharges _____

Nosocomial infections initially detected by:
  Inpatient surveillance
  Follow-up in
    a. Emergency department
    b. Outpatient department
    c. Other

	Number	% of total
	_____	_____
	_____	_____
	_____	_____
	_____	_____
Total	_____	100%

Ward or floor	Number of discharges	Number of infections	Attack rate, %	Service	Number of discharges	Number of infections	Attack rate, %
				Medicine			
				General surgery			
				Orthopedics			
				Urology			
				Other surgery subspecialty*			
				Gynecology			
				Obstetrics			
				Pediatrics			
				Newborn			
				Psychiatry			
				Other			

*Includes neurosurgery, ophthalmology, ENT, dental, and plastic surgery.

Figure 2
MONTHLY REPORT OF NOSOCOMIAL INFECTIONS

Pathogen	Site											
	Urinary tract		Respiratory		Surgical wounds	Burns	Other cutaneous	Gastro-intestinal	Genital	CNS	Blood	Other	Total
	Asympto-matic	Sympto-matic	Upper	Lower									
Alcaligenes													
Bacteroides													
Candida													
Citrobacter													
Clostridia													
D. pneumoniae													
Enterobacter													
Escherichia coli													
Enteropathogenic E. coli													
Hemophilus influenza													
Herellea													
Klebsiella													
Proteus mirabilis													
Proteus, other species													
Providencia													
Pseudomonas aeruginosa													
Pseudomonas, other species													
Salmonella													
Serratia													
Shigella													
Staphylococcus aureus													
Staphylococcus epidermidis													
Streptococcus group A, D, and other													
Streptococcus pneumoniae													
Streptococcus other													
Other bacterial pathogens													
Other pathogens													
No pathogens isolated													
Culture not done													

Figure 3

MONTHLY REPORT OF NOSOCOMIAL PATHOGENS AND SITES

- Maintain a continuing record (individual infection form or line listing) of each infection appearing after admission. Record the severity* of the infection, and update the record whenever indicated during the follow-up period. Maintain a close follow-up as indicated by severity of infection.
- Check necropsy reports to learn whether previously undiagnosed infection was found at autopsy.
- Maintain close liaison with the employee health service to ascertain the presence of infection in hospital personnel.
- Review all infection data at least weekly with the chairman of the infection control committee and/or the hospital epidemiologist; be particularly alert for clusters of infection.
- Prepare a monthly report of statistical data (Figure 2, page 24) for the infection control committee, staff physicians, and head nurses.
- Attend infection control committee meetings; submit the work sheets (Figure 1, page 22) to the committee for final classification and evaluation of postadmission infection.
- Establish a follow-up surveillance of discharged patients if the infection control committee so instructs.
- Record daily the number and type of infections present on admission of patients.

Control and Prevention

- Observe aseptic techniques; serve as consultant on isolation procedures.
- Consult on placement of patients with infections or patients with increased susceptibility to infection.
- Observe procedures for decontaminating equipment; provide assistance for microbiological examination of equipment when indicated.
- Participate in inservice education programs.
- Initiate, in consultation with the hospital epidemiologist, such studies as are indicated by the surveillance data.

An infection control nurse can carry out the duties outlined above in about 10 hours per week for each 100 beds. To maintain this program, the infection control nurse should limit activities to observing and recording ward events and abstracting information from patients' records for the infection control committee. The nurse should have authority to obtain necessary cultures on patients with suspect infections.

---

*†, minimal; ††, moderate; †††, serious; ††††, life threatening.

The success of such a surveillance program depends greatly upon the degree to which its purposes are explained to and clarified for the entire hospital staff. The hospital administration, infection control committee, and medical and nursing staffs must recognize that the ultimate goal of a surveillance program is the improvement of patient care.

EMPLOYEE HEALTH SERVICE

Because the hospital infection control program is designed to protect both patients and personnel, the hospital should provide for the detection, evaluation, prevention, and treatment of infection in its personnel.

Large hospitals might find it advantageous to establish an employee health service in a separate area of the hospital or in its clinics. In small hospitals with few full-time employees, this may not be economical or even feasible. However, whatever the size of the hospital, a physician and a nurse, on a full-time or a part-time basis, should be responsible for the health care of hospital personnel who become ill or are injured while on duty. Employees should be encouraged to report all job-related injuries to the employee health service. Procedures for the handling of emergency medical and surgical needs of employees should be known to all. A policy should be formulated regarding protection of unusually susceptible personnel, particularly those who are pregnant.

Medical Examination of Prospective Employees

All applicants for hospital employment should have an initial medical history and physical examination, chest x-ray, serologic test for syphilis, and tuberculin skin test. Follow-up skin testing of tuberculin-negative personnel should be carried out at least once each year. Tuberculin-positive personnel should be checked by an annual chest x-ray.

The immune status of new employees should be evaluated at the initial examination, and any necessary immunizations provided (see Immunization of Personnel, page 29).

In performing initial examinations, the employee health service must provide those examinations required by local or state health department regulations. Certain additional examinations, unless specifically required by local or state regulation, may best be left on an optional basis. For example, examination of food handlers for salmonella, shigella, or amoebic infections is not warranted as a general recommendation, but may be appropriate in hospitals located in areas where the endemic frequency of one or more of these diseases is high.

The epidemiologic significance of hepatitis B antigenemia is currently under active study. At this time, routine screening of hospital employees is not recommended.

Treatment of Personnel

Hospitals have not only the responsibility of protecting their personnel against acquiring infection from patients but also the responsibility of protecting patients from acquiring infection from hospital personnel. Thus, all personnel with illnesses should report to their supervisors or directly to the employee health service. Personnel who have direct or indirect contact with patients via food or fomites should be excused from duty if they have an infection that poses a hazard to patients or to other personnel. Such infections most commonly are those of the respiratory tract, the gastrointestinal tract, or the skin.

Appropriate therapy is the responsibility of the employee health service. Personnel who develop infections should be transferred to duties without direct patient contact or should be given leave with pay until they are no longer considered hazardous to others. In order to encourage reporting of infection by personnel, care must be taken that employees are in no way penalized by doing so.

Management of infection in hospital personnel calls for the exercise of thoughtful judgment. Patient care personnel having overt clinical infection, such as streptococcal pharyngitis, acute influenza, or a staphylococcal furuncle, should be restricted from patient contact. However, hospital personnel often experience minor infections of the skin, viral upper respiratory tract infections, and other areas. Personnel with such minor infections should report them to the health department and may usually continue to work so long as they have been clearly instructed about their potential risk to others and are scrupulous in their practice of personal hygiene. The nurse or the physician who is recovering from salmonellosis, for example, and who is still excreting salmonellae, usually need not be restricted from patient contact if good standards of personal hygiene are observed.

Prophylatic therapy should be provided to employees under certain circumstances, such as the use of gamma globulin after intimate exposure to hepatitis A; antibacterial therapy after intimate exposure to meningococcal meningitis (for example, mouth-to-mouth resuscitation attempts or accidents in the pipetting of spinal fluid); and tetanus toxoid booster immunizations following occupational injuries, unless the employee is already fully immunized.

Immunization of Personnel

Immunization against certain diseases should be made available for all hospital personnel through the employee health service. The type of immunization should be selected on the basis of risk. Records of the immunization status of hospital personnel must be kept by the employee health service.

Active immunization

The following active immunizations are recommended:

- *BCG.* The use of BCG *(bacille Calmette-Guérin)* vaccine for tuberculin-negative personnel in patient-contact positions should be considered in hospitals serving populations in which the endemic incidence of tuberculosis is high and the hospital employee tuberculin conversion rate is greater than one per cent each year for those employed in a specific department or service (see Appendix C, page 171).
- *Diphtheria-tetanus.* All personnel should be immunized against diphtheria and tetanus. Because diphtheria occurs most commonly in children, personnel most frequently in contact with sick children should maintain a high level of immunity. If reimmunization is offered to these personnel, the adult type of combined diphtheria-tetanus (Td) preparation should be given every 10 years.
- *Influenza.* Employees with a history of chronic cardiovascular or bronchopulmonary disease should be vaccinated against influenza each fall. In view of the increased safety and potency of influenza vaccines, vaccination of all hospital personnel is recommended, especially in anticipation of expected high incidence of influenza.
- *Measles (rubeola).* Nonpregnant women in the childbearing years who are employed in pediatric care and who have not had measles should be urged to accept immunization with a live measles vaccine.
- *Mumps.* Active immunization with live attenuated mumps vaccine is recommended for hospital personnel who have no history of clinical mumps.
- *Poliomyelitis.* Immunization against poliomyelitis should be offered to all personnel in accordance with current recommendations.
- *Rubella (German measles).* Female employees in the childbearing age range who may be exposed to rubella in the line of duty, who are unlikely to become pregnant within two months of vaccination, and who demonstrate no antibodies should be urged to accept rubella vaccination.

- *Smallpox.* All hospital personnel having contact with patients should receive smallpox vaccine upon employment and every three years thereafter. This procedure is particularly important in metropolitan areas.

Most outbreaks of smallpox in Western Europe have been in hospitals receiving patients from areas where smallpox is endemic. Prevention of smallpox in hospital personnel is especially important in relation to community protection. The appearance of smallpox in a hospital requires the vaccination or revaccination of all patients and personnel who have been exposed. Vaccinia immune globulin (VIG) should be given simultaneously with smallpox vaccine to exposed persons with the following conditions: eczema and other forms of chronic dermatitis; pregnancy; altered immune states such as leukemia, lymphoma, and other reticulo-endothelial malignancies; dysgammaglobulinemia; therapy with immunosuppressive drugs such as steroids and antimetabolites; or ionizing radiation.

Passive immunization

In addition to the immunizations already mentioned, passive immunization with immune globulin (gamma globulin) should be considered for the following kinds of exposure:

- *Hepatitis.* Persons who have had parenteral inoculation with needles or instruments accidentally contaminated with blood from a patient with hepatitis A or accidental fecal-oral exposure should be given immune serum globulin (human ISG) intramuscularly. A dosage of 0.01 milliliter per pound of body weight should be administered as soon as possible after the injury. Currently available ISG does not appear to protect against hepatitis B.
- *Poliomyelitis.* Administration of immune serum globulin to nonimmunized employees and patients who are exposed to an individual with poliomyelitis is not recommended. Unless previously immunized, individuals in contact with a poliomyelitis patient should receive an attenuated poliomyelitis vaccine (APV).
- *Smallpox and complications of vaccinia.* Special hyperimmune gamma globulin specific for vaccinia and smallpox has been shown to be of value in the management of complications of vaccinations.
- *Varicella-zoster.* Administration of zoster immune globulin should be considered for nonimmune persons who have had close exposure to varicella and who have impaired cell-mediated immunity.

Monitoring of Personnel

In general, routine programs designed to detect carriers of pathogens among hospital personnel contribute little to infection control. Programs to detect asymptomatic carriers of staphylococci, streptococci, meningococci, salmonellae, shigellae, and amoebae, therefore, are not recommended as a routine practice.

Outbreaks of infections within the hospital due to such organisms may prompt a search for personnel carriers as part of the study and control of the outbreak. The employee health service should assist in searches for carriers whenever indicated by specific epidemiologic circumstances.

EMPLOYEE EDUCATION PROGRAMS

In addition to providing an adequate employee health service, the hospital should establish educational programs for its personnel. These programs should thoroughly orient all hospital employees to the nature of nosocomial infections and to ways of preventing or controlling them.

If hospital personnel are to participate effectively in infection control programs, they must understand both the problem as it affects their work and the techniques necessary to function safely and properly. It is important that they be oriented and trained carefully and thoroughly.

Unfortunately, this is not a simple matter, because the transmission of infection from reservoir to host is often complex. In the hospital there are several potential reservoirs, including personnel, patients, and the hosts themselves. Furthermore, many of the organisms responsible for disease may be carried in an asymptomatic, or "silent," state. Personnel may find it difficult to comprehend this concept and to realize that, although they may be feeling entirely well, they may be a hazard to other persons.

The classical model for the transmission of infection is shown in Figure 4, next page.

The purpose of an educational program is to provide the information necessary to minimize factors favoring transmission of bacteria to susceptible patients. Most types of serious infection are transmitted by close contact between persons; however, it is obviously impossible to provide adequate patient care without close contact. Thus, personal hygiene becomes of paramount importance. Furthermore, proper measures must be undertaken to prevent contamination of patients or personnel from the environment.

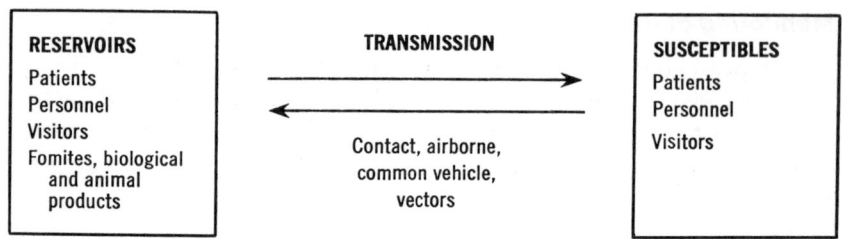

Figure 4
PATTERNS OF TRANSMISSION OF INFECTIONS IN THE HOSPITAL

Not all hospital personnel require the same degree of instruction with regard to nosocomial infection; hence the program for each category of personnel must be suited to the functional requirements of the work they perform. Failure of orientation and inservice training programs in infection control usually comes from inadequately adapting the program to the particular group or discipline to be reached.

Most hospital personnel belong to one of the following categories: administrative and office staff; medical staff, including attending physicians, house staff, and medical students; nursing personnel, including student and practical nurses and such others as attendants, aides, and orderlies; laboratory and autopsy room personnel; dietary staff, including dietitians, cooks, waitresses, and other workers; maintenance staff, including plumbers, steam fitters, and carpenters; and housekeeping and laundry personnel.

Because it is not possible to design a single orientation or inservice training program for these varied categories, consideration must be given to the specific problems and hazards pertinent to each category. The broad goals of the educational program, however, are similar for all hospital personnel, and in each instance should be designed to:

- Provide an understanding of the basic concepts of infection.
- Provide a working knowledge of the hazards associated with a particular category of employment.
- Convince each employee that he has a personal responsibility and role in the control of infection within the hospital.
- Provide a continuing educational program related to control of nosocomial infection.
- Reduce the hazard of acquired infection for each patient and employee.

One effective way to plan an education program is through the development of programmed methods of instruction. Specialized programs would be useful for personnel in the nursery, surgery, dietary department, and other services. This method of instruction would satisfy the information needs of personnel who represent different disciplines and who possess various levels of knowledge.

Although the type of instruction and particular examples used for illustration will differ substantially between, for example, the medical staff and laundry staff, the principles to be covered are similar and include information concerning the kinds and characteristics of organisms most likely to be of concern; the sources of these organisms; the epidemiological characteristics of nosocomial infection; the practice of aseptic techniques, hand washing, isolation, and special procedures for care of patients with infectious diseases; and the practice of decontamination, disinfection, and sterilization procedures.

The educational program might include the following specific elements: orientation program, procedure manuals, inservice training programs, and informal monitoring.

Orientation Program

A formal introduction to the hospital through an orientation program should be provided for new personnel in all categories. This program should include a description of the responsibility of the hospital and an overall view of the functions of the various departments. In addition to introducing the individual to the hospital itself, one of the goals of the orientation program should be an introduction to the principles and methods for the control of infection within the employee's particular department.

Procedure Manuals

Written procedure manuals for various departments are important for efficient operation. Specific procedures for the control of infection should be included in the manuals. Updated as necessary, manuals should be readily available to personnel working in the various departments.

Inservice Training Programs

An important part of the regular staff meetings of various hospital departments should be training programs devoted to descriptions of new infection control techniques or procedures useful to members of that particular department. The infection control nurse should participate in this activity. Meetings should also include a review of current hospital problems, with special reference to the role of the department in the genesis or control of these problems. A specific example or a cluster of cases may illustrate a point much more clearly than hours of formal presentation.

An educational program for hospital personnel must approach the problem of infection control in a way that is understandable to the individual employee and that will provide the practical and useful information needed to reduce hazards. The key features of any educational program of this type are practicality, attention to current problems, and research for more effective ways to provide greater safety for patients and personnel. Such a program has been developed by the Hospital Research and Educational Trust. Entitled *Team Up to Control Infection,* it consists of a coordinator's guide, supervisor's guide, and workers' books that accompany a film depicting a model program for hospital housekeeping personnel.

Informal Monitoring

The educational training of employees can often be augmented through informal monitoring. Observant personnel sometimes notice novice employees' breaks in technique, errors in equipment handling, and other potentially harmful practices. If these deficiencies in performance can be tactfully discussed at the time of occurrence, they can represent a useful form of inservice training.

Bacteriologic study before and after various types of cleaning, a demonstration of the values of various types of indicators in sterile packs, and similar procedures offer opportunities for supervisors to draw attention to problems of infection control.

REGULATIONS FOR HOSPITAL VISITORS

Because visitors may be sources of infection, suitable regulations pertaining to visitors are imperative in the control of nosocomial infection. Regulations governing the various services, as well as overall hospital policy, must be formulated with the collaboration and concurrence of the services concerned. Local customs, past experiences, and the structure of the hospital itself will influence the specific regulations.

Visiting patients is, basically, a privilege. Visiting often has therapeutic value—or the converse—and hence should be subject to the control of the attending physician. The rules and regulations regarding visiting should take into consideration such aspects as the areas of special risks of infection, the particular needs of individual patients, and the peak work periods of the staff. Certain patients may require special considerations, so visiting regulations should permit flexibility at the discretion of the attending physician.

General Considerations

The following list may be used as a guide in establishing policies for visitors.

Persons to exclude. Persons with respiratory disease or any signs of communicable infection should not be permitted to visit hospital patients. The age limit for admitting children varies; some hospitals permit children of 10 or 12 years to enter, but other hospitals permit only children more than 15 years of age.

Areas to be excluded. Visitors should not be permitted in the newborn nursery, operating rooms, or surgical recovery rooms. They should not be allowed in obstetrical delivery rooms or intensive care units unless strict controls are exercised.

Visiting hours. Preferably, visiting hours should not be scheduled during peak work periods of the hospital staff. However, for individual patients visiting hours may be varied by the attending physicians. Generally, two well-spaced two-hour visits will suffice, but some hospitals prefer a continuous visiting period from 11 a.m. to 8 p.m.

Behavior of visitors. Visitors must not interfere with the activities of the professional staff. Quiet should be maintained, and smoking should be restricted. Visitors should not bring food to patients unless specially advised to do so. They should not congregate in patient care areas and must not sit on patients' beds.

Number of visitors. Visiting privileges should be restricted primarily to family members. Preferably, there should be no more than two or three visitors per patient at any one time.

Protection of visitors. Information handouts on visiting regulations should be provided. Facilities and materials for protecting visitors from infected patients should be supervised and controlled by the nursing department.

Special Considerations

Certain areas require stricter control because of the greater hazards and more serious results of infections, and other areas may have special needs for visitors.

Pediatrics. Unlimited visiting privileges for mothers have been well accepted by the staff in many hospitals. This practice results in greater comfort and security for the child; it may also free the nursing staff from some of the more routine and time-consuming duties, because feeding, changing linen and clothing, and entertaining can be done by the mother. In some hospitals beds have been provided for mothers to remain in children's rooms on a full-time basis.

Newborn unit. No visitors should be permitted in the nursery, and infants should be viewed from the corridor during visiting hours only. Strict curtailment of visiting privileges is necessary with rooming-in care. If the infant is kept continuously at the mother's bedside, visiting should be restricted to only one person at a time. Only the mother and father should be permitted to handle the infant, since additional contact will increase the possibility of infection. With intermittent rooming-in care, visitors may be permitted in the mother's room during visiting hours while the infant is in the nursery. It is preferable in this situation for the mother to meet her visitors in a solarium or lounge if at all possible. With intermittent or continuous nursery care, the number of visitors need not be restricted as much as with rooming-in.

Burn treatment, isolation, and special-care areas. The number of visitors should be restricted, and visits should be limited to a few minutes. Visitors should be closely supervised and must avoid direct contact. Gowns and masks for visitors are advisable, unless visiting is done through windows. The patient and the visitor should be warned of the potential hazard of infection and the need for medical asepsis. Traffic in burn care areas must be restricted as much as possible. Visiting in all special care facilities, such as those for organ transplant or cancer chemotherapy or other areas where patients with extreme susceptibility to infection are located, should be similarly limited.

Operating rooms and recovery rooms. Nonprofessional visitors should not be allowed in operating rooms; nor should casual professional visitors be allowed, except in observation areas separated from the operating room by glass partitions. Nonprofessional visitors should not be permitted in recovery rooms. A husband may visit his wife in the labor or delivery room, if the policy for this has been established by the medical staff, if the facilities are suitable for this purpose, and if the visit is authorized by both the patient and the attending physician. Nonprofessional visitors in intensive care areas should be allowed only under strict controls.

BIBLIOGRAPHY

MEDICOLEGAL RESPONSIBILITIES

Edelman, J. *Darling v. Charleston Community Memorial Hospital*—How to adapt to the Charleston decision. *Mod. Hosp.* 107:137, Oct. 1966.

Hayt, E. Legal considerations in control of hospital infections. *Hospitals, J.A.H.A.* 50:75, Oct. 16, 1966.

Health Law Center. *Hospital Law Manual.* 2 vols. Pittsburgh: Aspen Systems Corp., 1959.

Hershey, N. What is legal duty in infection control? *Mod. Hosp.* 105:87, July 1965.

Hicks, J. T. Hospital acquired infections. *Hosp. Manage.* 105:47, Feb. 1968.

Horty, J. F. What the Charleston case means to hospitals. *Mod. Hosp.* 105:36, Dec. 1965.

INFECTION CONTROL COMMITTEE

American Public Health Association. *Control of Infectious Diseases in General Hospitals.* New York: APHA, 1967.

Association Section. Bulletin No. 1—Prevention and control of staphylococcus infections in hospitals. *Hospitals, J.A.H.A.* 32:49, July 1, 1958.

Joint Commission on Accreditation of Hospitals. *Accreditation Manual for Hospitals.* Chicago: JCAH, 1973.

MacIntosh, O. C. Defining "hospital infections." *Postgrad. Med.* 42:A119, Nov. 1967.

SURVEILLANCE AND REPORTING PROGRAMS

Brachman, P. S. Surveillance of hospital-associated infections. In: Williams, R. E. O., and Shooter, R. A., editors. *Infection in Hospitals: Epidemiology and Control.* Philadelphia: F. A. Davis Co., 1963, pp. 329-38.

Davis, N. C., and others. Infection control sister: her role in a large hospital. (Australia) *Lancet.* 2:1321, Dec. 21, 1963.

Eickhoff, T. C., and others. Surveillance of nosocomial infections in community hospitals. *J. Infect. Dis.* 120:305, Sept. 1969.

Gardner, A. M. N., and others. Infection control sister: a new member of the control of infection team in general hospitals. (UK) *Lancet.* 2:710, Oct. 6, 1962.

Lyon, P. Infection control nurse in a general hospital. *Can. Nurs.* 64:44, Jan. 1968.

Starkey, H. Surveillance of communicable infections in a hospital. *Can. Hosp.* 39:37, Nov. 1962.

EMPLOYEE HEALTH SERVICE

American Hospital Association and Center for Disease Control. *National Program for the Vaccination of Hospital Workers Against Smallpox.* Chicago: AHA, 1971.

American Hospital Association and American Medical Association. *Guiding Principles for an Occupational Health Program in a Hospital Employee Group.* Chicago: AMA, 1968.

Guidelines for immunization of hospital personnel. Center for Disease Control. *National Nosocomial Infections Study Quarterly Report.* First Quarter 1973 (in preparation).

Holland, P. V., and others. Gamma globulin in the prophylaxis of post-transfusion hepatitis. *J. Amer. Med. Assn.* 196:471, May 9, 1968.

Jones, T. O., and others. Viral hepatitis: a staff hazard in dialysis units. *Lancet.* 1:853, Apr. 1, 1967.

Shu, C. Y. Smallpox vaccination of hospital personnel urged. *Hospitals, J.A.H.A.* 47:95, Dec. 1, 1973.

Smallpox (Editorial). *Brit. Med. J.* 1:288, Feb. 10, 1951.

Wehrle, P. F. The risk of poliomyelitis infection among exposed hospital personnel. *J. Pediat.* 17:237, Feb. 1956.

Wehrle, P. F., and others. An airborne outbreak of smallpox in a German hospital and its significance with respect to other recent outbreaks in Europe. *Bull. WHO.* 43:669, 1970.

EMPLOYEE EDUCATION PROGRAMS

Hospital Research and Educational Trust. *Programmed Instruction and the Hospital.* Chicago: HRET, 1967.

──────────────. *Team Up To Control Infection.* Chicago: HRET, 1973.

Koren, H. Self-inspection program raises cleanliness level. *Hospitals, J.A.H.A.* 42:107, Feb. 16, 1968.

Mallison, G. F. Audiovisual aids on hospital sanitation and institutional infections. *J. Environ. Health.* 29:64, July-Aug. 1966.

Parisi, J. T. Teaching infection control methods to ancillary service personnel. *Hospitals, J.A.H.A.* 42:82, Mar. 16, 1968.

Seedor, M. M. *Introduction to Asepsis, Programmed Unit in Fundamentals of Nursing.* Rev. ed. New York City: Teachers College, Columbia University, 1964.

Chapter 4

Specific Responsibilities Within Hospitals

Prevention and control of nosocomial infection demands more than the existence of an active infection control committee and an informed and conscientious staff. Specific responsibilities must be assigned, both to individuals and to departments, for effective infection control.

CORPORATE RESPONSIBILITIES

The health care institution as an entity has an overall responsibility for assessment, prevention, and control of infection within its premises. The governing body and all other component parts of the institution thus retain a legitimate continuing interest in this problem.

INDIVIDUAL RESPONSIBILITIES

Those individuals with the greatest responsibility are the administrator, the physician, the epidemiologist, and the nurse.

The Administrator

The hospital administrator has broad responsibilities in the prevention and control of nosocomial infections.

He must provide adequate microbiological services and facilities. He must budget judiciously to meet the financial requirements of the infection control program. He must also publicize and implement this program by providing for the orientation of all personnel, by creating concern for the prevention of infection, and by placing special emphasis on the importance of sterilization and disinfection techniques. He must establish regulations for visitors, inspect hospital conditions, and evaluate practices in conjunction with the infection control program. In addition, he must provide administrative representation on the infection control committee and ensure the participation of various hospital departments in the activities of this committee.

It is the administrator's responsibility to delegate authority to the nursing service for the isolation of patients with overt contagious diseases until these patients have been examined by a physician. He must ensure the establishment and maintenance of a mechanism for prompt and complete reporting of infectious and communicable diseases both to the infection control committee and to the health department. He must make sure that every effort is made to provide compensation and care for personnel who develop potentially communicable infections (see Infected Personnel and Carriers, page 119).

The administrator should ensure continued liaison with the local health department and with other agencies concerned with infection control. He may function as the chief public relations authority for the release of news items or medical information; if he delegates this responsibility, he must maintain constant surveillance over the public release of such information.

The Physician

The physician has major responsibilities in the prevention and control of nosocomial infections, such as exercising his patient care duties, serving as a member of the infection control committee, functioning as a hospital epidemiologist or infection control officer, and setting a good example in the practice of medical asepsis. In short, the physician can best discharge his responsibilities by continuously striving to create and to maintain barriers between the patient and the pathogenic microorganisms within the hospital.

Because of his awareness of the patient's susceptibility to nosocomial infection, the physician should attempt to limit exposure of his patient to potentially pathogenic bacteria and viruses. A basic preventive measure is protecting his patient from hospital personnel who may be infected and from other patients with apparent infection. Moreover, the physician has the responsibility to prevent transfer of infection from his patient to other patients or to staff members. The physician must insist on proper hand washing by everyone whose duties require personal contact with his patient and also on the utilization of reverse isolation when indicated.

The physician can exert effective leadership in the promotion of medical asepsis through his precept and example. When the physician constantly employs all proper safeguards against the transmission of infection while in contact with patients himself, he is in a position to set an excellent example for other hospital personnel. This is particularly true in the case of such routine and often neglected procedures as hand washing.

Specific measures. The physician can increase his effectiveness in infection control by: (1) gaining thorough familiarity with the practices and procedures recommended by the infection control committee and closely adhering to them; (2) ordering cultures to detect the presence and determine the identity of bacteria suspected of causing infection; (3) reporting nosocomial infection to the hospital infection committee; (4) alerting the hospital of the pending admission of an infected patient; (5) acting according to the recommendations of the committee concerning limitations on the use of antibacterial agents for systemic administration; (6) instructing patients, relatives of patients, and hospital personnel in techniques for preventing the spread of infection; and (7) reporting and instituting appropriate treatment for any infection appearing in himself, and taking appropriate measures to avoid the possibilities of transmitting such infection to patients.

Service on the infection control committee. As a member of the infection control committee, the physician can apply his knowledge of infectious disease and its containment on an institutionwide basis. Thus he will concern himself with reporting of infections, analyzing reports of infection, solving housekeeping problems, training personnel, analyzing the use of antibiotics and adrenocortical steroids, and developing immunization programs. He will be concerned with admission policies, aseptic procedures in the various departments of the hospital, discipline of personnel, effectiveness of the bacteriology laboratory, and hepatitis screening of prospective blood donors. As a committee member, the physician's responsibilities require a performance beyond the usual call of duty, for he functions as an agent for all the physicians who admit patients to the hospital as well as for the patients themselves.

The Epidemiologist

One person who can be especially helpful to the infection control committee is the hospital epidemiologist, or the infection control officer. This position must be filled by someone interested in infections, committed to surveillance, and knowledgeable in epidemiology and biostatistics. The main qualifications of the hospital epidemiologist are interest, available time, and a sense of responsibility.

The individual must be a member of the infection control committee, possibly its chairman. The epidemiologist and the infection control nurse, who works under the epidemiologist's immediate direction, represent the infection control committee; they carry out the recommendations of the committee and conduct investigations.

The immediate concerns of the epidemiologist might include such matters as: (1) adequacy of the infection reporting system; (2) investigation of infectious diseases occurring within the hospital; (3) evaluation of the adequacy of isolation procedures; (4) sanitation; (5) sterilization; (6) employee health programs; and (7) collection and analysis of data on such considerations as promiscuous use of antimicrobial agents, incidence of hepatitis following transfusions, and incidence of urinary infection following catheterization.

The epidemiologist should act as the liaison officer between the hospital and the local health department, be concerned with the occurrence of employee infections that *may* have resulted from patient contacts, and assist in the development of educational programs for employees. Such functions are best served by a physician who has been trained in epidemiology. Some hospitals promote this kind of expertise by appointing staff physicians to take courses in epidemiology and to serve as part-time epidemiologists.

The Nurse

Carrying out the practical aspects of infection control is largely a function of the nursing service staff, who handle not only routine matters but special needs as well. Nurses must know how to perform all the procedures necessary for the prevention or containment of infection. They serve as sources of information for others and carry out special supervisory and reporting duties. Many of their duties and responsibilities are both burdensome and exacting and demand careful planning and programming. As nurses are the only persons in the hospital close to the patient every hour of the day and night, only they can provide continuous professional supervision with respect to infection control.

Although nursing responsibilities rest primarily on the registered nurse, all other members of the nursing service share these responsibilities to the extent of their training and the nature of their assigned duties. Included among these other nursing service personnel are licensed practical nurses, nursing aides, operating room technicians, and orderlies.

The responsibilities of the nursing service can be considered in these categories: the administrative nurse (director of nursing and supervisory staff), the practicing nurse (nursing unit staff), the infection control nurse, and the public health nurse. These responsibilities can be shifted from one nurse to another as organizational circumstances require.

The administrative nurse

The administrative nurse has a professional obligation to actively support and participate as a member in the deliberations of the infection control committee, bringing to the committee essential information and important suggestions. The nurse can also help to develop and implement procedures and practices for the nursing service that best fit into the general framework of the infection control program.

The administrative nurse should develop training programs on infection control for all new nursing department employees and should be available for consultation with other department heads to help orient their personnel to asepsis and to other techniques important in infection control. The nurse should also be available for planning and supervising infection control procedures in such specialized areas as surgery, newborn nursery, intensive care unit, and central sterile supply. Service as an adviser should help in maintaining interest and morale with respect to infection control measures among nursing personnel.

The administrative nurse may be of assistance when differences of opinion arise between physicians and nurses. Such differences should be brought to the attention of the infection control committee. Constant review of the entire nursing program as it applies to infection control and the elimination of any outmoded or unnecessary procedures are other functions of the administrative nurse. Finally, an infection control program can be effective only if the administrative nurse and the supervisory staff provide firm support.

The practicing nurse

The practicing nurse is responsible for all nursing functions essential in the prevention, recognition, and management of infection. A practicing nurse needs thorough familiarity with the infection control program in order to support all its policies, practices, and procedures. Regular attention to measures of medical asepsis, including handwashing and isolation techniques, is a most important responsibility. The nurse should be constantly alert to report signs of infection such as fever, chills, shock, cellulitis, pus, and diarrhea in patients.

Through careful recording in nursing notes, as well as through notices to the physician, nursing supervisor, and infection control committee, the practicing nurse is a basic source of information on infections.

The hospital procedures should include authority for the nurse to take appropriate interim action upon signs of infectious disease potentially hazardous to others. It is recommended that hospitals have standing orders that permit nurses to effectuate interim isolation of and to take cultures on patients who are admitted with or who develop communicable infectious disease.

The practicing nurse can protect patients against exposure to infection from visitors, from hospital staff, from other patients and their fomites, and from materials and equipment used in diagnosis and treatment. The nurse can also serve as an instructor and supervisor for subordinate personnel, patients, and visitors in matters of personal hygiene, aseptic techniques, and the like. The nurse's participation in new infection control techniques and procedures will help in the realistic evaluation of them.

The infection control nurse

Administrative arrangements for appointing an infection control nurse vary among hospitals, depending upon local considerations. It is desirable to assign a nurse who has particular interests and capabilities in infection control. The establishment of such a position represents an advance in infection control, and the position undoubtedly is one that hospitals should establish, if only on a part-time basis.

The infection control nurse must be not only knowledgeable but also tactful, considerate, and known to and respected by the hospital staff. Training in epidemiology, surveillance, and basic statistical methods is necessary.

At the discretion of the infection control committee, the authorization of the infection control nurse should cover such duties as case finding, surveillance and reporting, analysis and interpretation, epidemic investigation, inspection, program evaluation and recommendation, control, education, and prevention. The infection control nurse routinely reports to and consults with the committee member who has been designated the hospital epidemiologist.

In addition to carrying out the surveillance and reporting duties listed on page 21, the infection control nurse can also serve as an observer of the general state of cleanliness, the skill used in practicing asepsis, isolation techniques, decontamination procedures, and other matters relating to infection control. The infection control nurse should also have the authority, after conferring with the patient's physician if available, to order or obtain cultures in all suspect infections, to put into action such control measures as isolation, and to take corrective actions whenever gross breaks in techniques occur that require prompt remedial action.

The efforts of the infection control nurse should not be restricted solely to infections in patients. The nurse should also keep aware of the health of employees, especially with respect to infections, and should teach hospital personnel how to protect themselves against acquiring infections in the course of their patient care duties. The nurse should also promote the immunization programs recommended by the American Medical Association and the American Hospital Association, and should be constantly concerned with follow-up procedures that will help employees to maintain their immunities at effective levels.

Many liaison functions between the infection control committee and the various departments of the hospital can be handled by the infection control nurse, who can also serve as a liaison between the hospital and community health authorities, including visiting nurses and public health nurses responsible for home care of discharged patients. Community health authorities can perform more effectively if the infection control nurse informs them of infection present in discharged patients. Public health nurses are also a source of information on infection in discharged patients.

The public health nurse

The hospital door is not an efficient microbial barrier. It allows anyone entering the hospital to bring infection in and permits discharged patients to carry nosocomial infection out to their families and to others in the community. Much good could be accomplished if physicians and hospitals would regularly utilize the services of the public health nurse, who can make significant contributions in reducing the spread of infection into and out of the hospital.

Whether a member of the local health department or of a voluntary agency such as the Visiting Nurse Association, the public health nurse can be helpful in a variety of ways. For example, when a patient with an infection is to be discharged from the hospital, the public health nurse could make preparations to carry out necessary treatments at home; initiate measures of asepsis to prevent the spread of infection to family and community; and report the patient's progress to the hospital's attending physician or the infection control nurse or both. In some situations, the public health nurse may be requested to maintain surveillance on susceptible discharged patients who did not have clinical disease at the time of discharge.

If such services are established through a good working relationship with the public health nurse, in many instances the attending physician and the hospital should be able to discharge patients with infection considerably earlier than is now possible. The economic importance of such an arrangement is easily recognized.

The public health nurse can be of considerable service in other ways. For example, if a patient to be discharged is free from infection but his physical condition makes him susceptible to infection (see Opportunistic Pathogens and the Compromised Host, page 10), the attending physician and the hospital may request evaluation of the home situation by the public health nurse. Through this nurse, measures can be instituted to improve the home environment; make it safer for the patient; and reduce the patient's exposure to infection, both in the hospital and after discharge, by discouraging visits from relatives and friends with active infection. However, the public health nurse cannot function independently; patient care services can be given only on the request of the attending physician.

DEPARTMENTAL RESPONSIBILITIES

Various departments also hold important responsibilities through their role in infection control. Among these departments are the microbiological laboratory, the pharmacy, central supply, food service, and those concerned with housekeeping and maintenance. Heads of these departments may find that reports of specific infection control activities are useful in directing staff attention to current problems.

The Microbiological Laboratory

Access to a dependable microbiological laboratory is essential not only for proper diagnosis and management of infection in patients but also as a resource for effective operation of the infection control program of the hospital. The laboratory must promptly report unusual microbiological results to the epidemiologist or to the chairman of the infection control committee.

The results of microbiologic studies are of such great importance to the infection control program that provision must be made for the centralized collection of data on: (1) etiology of infections and the results of follow-ups on patients and members of the staff, (2) presence of unusual or hazardous microorganisms, (3) results of serological, bacteriological, and parasitological examinations of hospital staff, and (4) results of routine checks and special studies on the adequacy of sterilization procedures.

In many hospitals, the laboratory accepts the responsibility of keeping these records for the infection control committee. As part of its infection control procedures, the laboratory staff identifies and records the number and types of microbial agents isolated from patients and from hospital personnel.

In any event, the laboratory personnel should be responsible for: (1) maintenance of current data on antibiotic sensitivity patterns for at least staphylococci and gram-negative microorganisms isolated from overt infections of clinical importance; (2) protection of laboratory personnel against occupational hazards; (3) liaison with public health or reference laboratories for quality control, for special laboratory procedures, and for reporting or identifying certain infectious agents, as required.

Areas of responsibility

It is necessary that the microbiological laboratory be planned, equipped, and staffed to handle two areas of responsibility: the microbiological diagnosis of patients and personnel and the implementation of safety measures to prevent the conveyance of infection to laboratory workers.

Hospital laboratories ordinarily are equipped and staffed for the identification of microorganisms and the support of a surveillance program. In some hospitals, phage typing, serological, or other specific identifications are done in the hospital's own laboratory; in other hospitals, these identifications are done in a public health laboratory or in a reference laboratory. In any case, two requirements essential for flexibility should be emphasized: avoidance of overloading senior supervisory personnel with routine commitments and establishment of active liaison with public health laboratories.

Much of the routine work supporting the surveillance programs consists of scheduled checks on the efficiency of sterilization (see Environmental Control, page 78). To support specific epidemiologic investigations or training exercises, the laboratory also should be familiar with standard methods for the sampling of medications, medical supplies, equipment, and other objects for microbial contamination.

In vitro trials of disinfectants and antiseptics are only rough guides to their activity. Their true efficacy can be assessed only by properly controlled inuse tests. Where the laboratory can perform these tests reliably, they may be useful in evaluating changes in materials or procedures. If false results from bacterial dormancy induced by residual chemical action are to be avoided, techniques to assess disinfectants must include provisions for the neutralization of residual activities of such substances on the test bacteria. Because of the difficulties in performing these tests, most hospitals are advised to consult standard references and authorities.

Implementing safety measures

Laboratory safety standards are a mutual responsibility of hospital management and the director of laboratory services. The details of planning and equipping individual laboratories vary in accordance with the scope and type of work undertaken, but certain principles must be borne in mind in all instances.

Routine bacteriological work always creates potential occupational hazards for technicians. Making direct smears on glass slides, flaming loops, or spreaders, removing cotton-wool plugs or caps from culture tubes, subculturing bacterial growths, and some methods of centrifuging create aerosols, or airborne particles. These contaminate the immediate surroundings of the technician and the technician's hands, clothes, and so forth. It follows that all work surfaces and floors must be cleaned frequently with suitable disinfectants; that bench and apparatus cleaning must be done by well-trained housekeeping staff; that technicians must wear protective, frequently changed smocks or uniforms; that the value of frequent, efficient hand washing must be stressed; and that working areas must not be subjected to discernible drafts or air currents.

If bacteria or viruses known to be particularly virulent or easily transmissible are to be handled in the laboratory, special provisions must be made. *Mycobacterium tuberculosis* is a particular hazard because it survives drying. Pasteurella, brucella, and psittacosis organisms have been transmitted to and have caused severe illness in laboratory personnel. These virulent agents must either be sent to some other specially equipped laboratory, or be handled by technicians using special procedures or techniques. These include wearing protective clothing; working in a specially designed, easily cleaned room; and conducting the procedures in sterilizable cabinets with glove ports.

Unidirectional, or laminar flow, units, or specially designed clean rooms or hoods with separate air exhaust systems, are also useful for this type of work. The efflux from the exhaust systems should be sterilized by heat or passed through high-efficiency filters. It is advisable to draw air into such a room from the next room or corridor through a filter, rather than to try to balance an air delivery and exhaust system for constant negative pressure in the room. Ventilation systems in microbiological laboratories should be so arranged that all corridors, offices, and noncontaminated rooms have slightly positive pressure, whereas all contaminated rooms have negative pressure.

Laboratory procedures involving clean materials or equipment should not be undertaken in an area used for contaminated material procedures. In order to prevent contamination of the hospital environment, laboratory animals should be located in a separate area or room. The arrangements should include facilities for technicians to wash and dress; for safe disposal of animals, their excreta, and other contaminated materials; and for dust control.

A number of regulations are required for the protection of the laboratory staff in general:

- All materials known to be contaminated must be clearly identified. Color-coded adhesive tape is a useful device to indicate contamination.
- When examinations and tests are completed, all hazardous materials must be sterilized before disposal.
- Identification, collection, delivery, and handling of specimens from all patients under isolation must be the subject of special regulations agreed upon by the infection control committee.
- All accidents in the laboratory involving potential hazards to personnel should be reported to the laboratory director immediately.

It should be noted that specimens from patients may convey infection to all types of laboratory staff, including those in hematology, pathology, and so forth. Routine procedures to protect staff from such agents as hepatitis viruses must be maintained.

The Pharmacy

The responsibilities of the pharmacy are:

- To dispense antimicrobial drugs. Reference data describing their actions, incompatibilities, and deteriorative characteristics should be on file and available on request, to be distributed with the prior approval of the pharmacy committee.
- To obtain, store, dispense, and distribute therapeutic materials in such a form that infective agents will not be conveyed to patients or to treatment facilities.
- To obtain, store, and make available for emergency use vaccines, serums, and other biological therapeutic materials.
- To maintain records, including lot numbers, of drugs and other materials dispensed for use in the hospital, in accordance with the requirements of physicians and with the regulations of the pharmacy and therapeutics committee.

- To consult the infection control committee regarding the use of certain antimicrobial agents and antisera.
- In accordance with hospital policy, to add medications to high-volume parenteral fluids, either through central service or satellite preparation stations.

In the implementation of the foregoing directives, the following is also essential. Procedures for dispensing sterile supplies through the pharmacy must be established as agreed upon by the infection control committee. In addition, sterile supplies must be stored and transported in such a manner as to prevent contamination by rough handling, puncturing of containers, or alterations of wrappings. As part of the infection control education program, users of sterile material should be made familiar with any peculiarities of either materials or containers that might lead to easy contamination. This is especially important in the case of intravenous solutions.

To prevent cross infection, single-dose or single-use containers should be dispensed whenever possible. If solutions, lubricants, or ointments are required for multiple use, preservatives or antibacterial agents should be incorporated in them. The staff should be informed about the hazards of bacterial conveyance from patient to patient or from staff to patient in such cases, and pertinent training procedures should be reviewed by the infection control committee.

All disinfectants, antiseptics, and other antibacterial substances purchased by and issued from the pharmacy should have the following data recorded for the information of the pharmacists and for the instruction of the users: (1) active properties relating to inuse strength, temperature, killing times, and microbes affected; (2) toxic, sensitizing, or other tissue-damaging qualities; (3) incompatible substances or materials, especially those that serve to weaken the agent; and (4) physical conditions, such as temperature, light, and moisture, that may adversely influence activity after storage. When feasible, undiluted solutions should be used to minimize chances of contamination during reconstitution to proper dilution.

The Central Supply Service

It is preferable that all equipment and supplies requiring special cleaning or sterilization be centrally handled whenever possible. Regardless of the organizational pattern of the hospital, the responsibility for the implementation of such central control must be specifically assigned. This responsibility includes receiving, processing, storing, and issuing various kinds of materials, such as items sterilized in the hospital, items purchased already sterile, and equipment requiring cleaning and repairing before reuse.

Specifications for the purchase of all items, whether disposable or not, should be established in consultation with the supervisor of central supply. Standard written procedures for all items pertinent to infection control should be adopted after approval by the infection control committee. All supplies and equipment to be used within patient care areas should be handled as if they were potential sources for transmitting infection.

Nonsterile materials

A facility for the receiving, servicing, cleaning, storing, and issuing of nonsterile equipment should be provided. This facility should handle such items as ward beds, special stands or tables, lamps, heaters, special chairs, and stretchers. Techniques and materials to be used for the cleaning of such equipment prior to reissue should be reviewed by the infection control committee. Particular attention should be given to the selection of disinfectants to be used.

Prepackaged and presterilized materials

Prepackaged and presterilized equipment, materials, or solutions should be stored and handled in a standardized manner by a single department. After definition by the prospective users, the specifications for purchase should be cleared through the infection control committee.

Sterile reusable materials

This service requires at least two physically separate areas: one for receipt and cleaning of dirty materials that will be reused and another for handling and storage of sterile materials. A third useful area would be one for handling and packaging of clean but not sterile materials.

The greatest emphasis should be placed on efficient washing and cleaning of equipment and materials such as tubing, valves, and rubber gloves. Automatic washing and rinsing machines should be used wherever possible, but a strict inspection system is still necessary. Ultrasonic tanks are particularly valuable for removal of dirt from equipment surfaces prior to the final washing.

Rigid standards must be established for packing and wrapping sets or items of equipment, the size or arrangement of packages, and the kind of wrapping materials or containers. The choices should be made on the basis of steam or disinfectant penetrability and on shelf-life maintenance of sterility. Reusable equipment and supplies should be purchased, so far as possible, on the basis of their reactions to steam or ethylene oxide sterilization. Chemical sterilization should be necessary only when it has been clearly established that no steam-resistant article is available for purchase (see Sterilization and Disinfection, page 93).

Sterile supplies

The storage and handling of sterile supplies must be planned to avoid gross contamination of the permeable wrappings of packaged materials. Standards must be established for the shelf life of different types of packages in terms of the expected contamination of the package surface and the likelihood of bacterial penetration of the wrappings.

Supplies properly wrapped in double-thickness permeable material comprising four layers can be expected to remain sterile for at least four weeks under normal conditions of clean storage. Protection against contamination of sterile, wrapped supplies depends mainly upon the porosity of the wrapper and the method of wrapping. Proper rotation of stock will reduce the need for resterilization. Addition of impermeable outer wrappings or placing of packages in metal containers may extend the shelf life of infrequently used materials up to six months. The storage area and the cupboards must be designed for easy washing; a schedule of frequent, careful cleaning must be maintained.

Sterile supplies must be transported in clean containers or carriers. The containers should not be the same as those used for the collection and return of contaminated materials unless they are washed and sterilized between trips.

The Food Service Department

The general responsibilities of the food service department are:
- To develop and maintain clean and sanitary work areas, storage areas, and equipment for the handling of supplies in accordance with state and local health department standards.
- To develop written standards and work procedures for daily operations. Procedures for preparation and serving of food must be such as to minimize contamination by microorganisms and chemicals that may result in food poisoning.
- To prepare purchasing specifications that meet the requirements of safety and sanitation for food, equipment, serviceware, and cleaning supplies.
- To develop procedures, and put them in writing, for cleaning and sanitizing trays and tableware after use in patient and personnel meal service. Service in isolation rooms should be planned in cooperation

with the infection control committee and the nursing service, and disposable materials should be used whenever possible.
- To develop procedures that comply with the local health department regulations for storage, handling, and disposal of garbage and refuse.
- To develop programs for the training of personnel in food preparation procedures and personal cleanliness and care, in compliance with regulations established by the infection control committee and the employee health service.

Written standards, work procedures, and cleaning schedules for the daily operation of the food service department are essential for effective management of the department. They also form the basis of training materials for food service personnel.

Many food service employees have little or no prior knowledge of sanitation requirements. It is necessary, therefore, to have a regularly scheduled training program for new personnel (see Orientation Program, page 33). Because the application of sanitary practice in food service requires constant vigilance, permanent employees may also benefit from periodic participation in the program. This program should emphasize employees' personal hygiene, including the importance of frequent and careful hand washing; procedures for reporting all infections, especially those of the skin, gastrointestinal and respiratory tracts; and descriptions of physical conditions and diseases prohibiting direct contacts with foods. At a minimum, food service employees who have had diarrheal disease should be free of salmonella and shigella before returning to work. The program should conform to local health department requirements. An explanation of the causes of food contamination and of the means of prevention, including the relationships of temperature to bacterial growth and sanitizing procedures, should be included to give personnel an understanding of the basis for approved food and equipment handling procedures.

General principles of protection

In protecting against the inception of nosocomial infection in food-handling areas, certain general principles should be kept in mind. Foremost is the fact that the foods most likely to be contaminated at the time of purchase are eggs, cream-filled pastries, and poultry. Fresh meats and fish should also be regarded as potentially contaminated. Federal or state certification of wholesome foods processed under sanitary conditions is required for fresh or processed foods containing meats, poultry, fish, eggs, milk, and other dairy foods.

The dietitian should make it a practice to visit periodically the sources of supply of such items in order to be assured that sanitary conditions prevail and to impress upon the vendors real concern about the possible contamination of foods. Cracked or checked eggs must not be purchased, because of the likelihood of salmonella contamination. Only pasteurized dairy products and pasteurized frozen or pasteurized powdered eggs should be purchased. Pasteurized frozen or pasteurized powdered eggs should be used only in dishes requiring prolonged heating, such as baked goods.

The crucial factors in the possible entry and growth of contaminants in all kinds of food are amount of hand contact, cleanliness of equipment, and length of time these foods are held between 7°C. (45°F.) and 60°C. (140°F.), other than during the necessary periods of preparation and service.

Equipment

Standards for design, construction, and maintenance of many types of equipment have been developed by the National Sanitation Foundation. Equipment that meets these standards may be stamped with the NSF seal of approval; this seal should be included in specifications for equipment purchased for the food service department.

Work areas and equipment should be designed and installed in accordance with recommendations of sanitary engineers, in order to ensure safe and adequate supplies of water, steam, power, or heat, as well as to enable easy cleaning. State and local health department regulations stipulate certain space and installation requirements as well as routine inspections of operation procedures. Specifications for tableware, small equipment, paper supplies, disposables, and cleaning supplies should also be developed to ensure standards of sanitation.

Federal and local health services have well-defined requirements for dishwashing equipment and dish-handling procedures. Representatives of manufacturers of dishwashing machines and compounds are available for training of food service personnel in these requirements. Personnel should be made aware of the need to furnish patients and personnel with properly sanitized trays and tableware as well as to protect themselves in the handling of soiled dishes.

Total disposable tray service is useful for patients in strict and enteric isolation. Use of disposable trays, dishes, plastic flatware, and packaged condiments permits incineration of these items and eliminates sterilization problems.

Storage

Arrangements and cleaning procedures for storage areas, to prevent contamination of stored foods and supplies by rodents, insects, and moisture, should be in compliance with state and local food establishment regulations.

Food storage refrigerators and freezers should be provided with thermometers to give assurance that foods are kept at appropriate temperatures. The ideal ranges are as follows: fruits and vegetables, dairy products, meat and poultry at temperatures from 7°C. (45°F.) to 0.5°C. (33°F.); fish and shellfish, ice cream, and frozen foods at temperatures from below freezing to −23.5°C. (−10°F.). Frozen food that has been thawed should not be refrozen, but should be used immediately afterward.

Shelf space for all foods should be provided with a floor clearance of 4 to 6 inches to permit proper floor cleaning.

Food preparation

Separate work areas should be assigned for the preparation of cold foods and hot foods. All work areas and equipment should be kept clean. Cooked foods should reach a temperature throughout of at least 74°C. (165°F.). Browning of meringue is not to be regarded as thorough cooking. Prior to use, raw fruits and vegetables must be washed under running water.

All foods should be kept covered between the time of preparation and the time of serving. Hot food should be held at 60°C. (140°F.) or higher, and cold foods at 7°C. (45°F.) or lower. Stuffings or dressings require thorough cooking because they are particularly likely to be vehicles for foodborne infection; they should be baked separately from poultry, never within the body cavity.

Food service

Service of foods requires the following precautions in order to safeguard the health of patients and staff:
- Food should be served as soon as possible after its preparation.
- Suitable utensils should be provided and used in order to reduce manual contact with food to a minimum. The same precautions apply to the handling of ice cubes.
- Individual portions of food not consumed by the patient should be discarded.
- In dishwashing machines all dishes must be washed in water at a temperature of 60°C. (140°F.) for 20 seconds and rinsed at a minimum temperature of 82°C. (180°F.) for 10 seconds. When dishes are

washed manually, they should be washed in water at a temperature of 43.5° to 49°C. (110° to 120°F.) with an adequate amount of soap or detergent, and then sanitized at 76.5°C. (170°F.) for at least half a minute in a solution containing an effective sanitizing agent.
- Employees with potentially communicable diseases, such as upper respiratory illness, skin infections, and enteric diseases, should not be allowed to handle food or equipment.
- Clean toilets and handwashing facilities should be provided convenient to food preparation areas. Installing the handwashing facility *outside* the toilet area, in an easily observed location, has been found to induce more use by the staff.

Any occurrence of food poisoning requires prompt reporting and immediate action to trace it back to the source of contamination; it also requires confirmation that the water and milk supplies have been checked periodically by the public health department and that the reports are satisfactory. All menus for patients and staff should be kept for a minimum of 30 days, as a possible aid in tracing a source of contamination.

Responsibilities of the director

To carry out his job, the director of food service should have a background that includes some knowledge of bacteriology, food procurement, personnel training, storage, food preparation, work analysis, departmental layouts, and equipment design and specifications. All these are essential if the director is to understand the general requirements of the food service department and be able to comply fully with them. If the person in charge of the food service department has not had this kind of educational background, the services of appropriate consultants or members of the medical staff should be made available for guidance and aid.

The Laundry and Linen Service

Soiled linen is a significant source of microbial contamination. Adequate procedures for the collection, transportation, processing, and storage of hospital linen are essential in order to eliminate the possibility of infection from this source.

Because of the potential hazards, all personnel who are in contact with soiled linen should be considered a risk. They should receive instructions on how to protect themselves and others.

Handling soiled linens

All soiled linen should be bagged at the location used. Linen should be removed from beds and handled with a minimum of agitation in order to prevent gross airborne microbial contamination. Blankets should be laundered after each patient's use. Mattresses should be enclosed with covers of impervious plastic in order to prevent contamination and to permit easy cleaning.

Soiled linen should not be sorted or prerinsed in patient care units. Linen should be removed at least daily from patient care units, and at least twice daily from nurseries; all nursery linen should be stored and transported in separate impervious bags.

Linen known to be contaminated with infectious microorganisms, particularly from isolation areas, should be clearly labeled and handled with special care. Impervious color-coded bags are recommended. Plastic bags soluble in hot water, which can be placed directly into washing machines, are excellent for use with isolation linen. Cloth bags for soiled linen require the same laundering as their contents.

All soiled linen should be transported in well-covered and clearly identified carts used exclusively for that purpose. The liners of these carts should be cleaned or laundered frequently. If chutes are used, all linen so transported should be bagged. Chutes should be cleaned on a regular schedule. All chute charging doors should be tight-fitting, self-closing, and located in separate, well-ventilated, fireproof rooms—not in corridors.

Soiled linen should be handled and sorted as little as possible. Rooms for storing and sorting soiled linen in the hospital laundry should be separate from other processing rooms. Ideally, they should be under negative pressure; and they should be ventilated with 10 room-volumes per hour directly to the outside, with no recirculation. The soiled linen area should be thoroughly cleaned and disinfected daily.

In addition to a storage and sorting room, separate rooms are required in the hospital laundry for processing, for clean storage and sewing, for toilet and handwashing facilities, and for an office. The laundry should be designed to handle seven days' load of soiled linen within the workweek. The flow of ventilation air in the laundry should be from the cleanest to the dirtiest areas. The floor and all equipment in the laundry should be cleaned at the end of each workday, and a regular schedule should be established and maintained to clean overhead and hard-to-wash areas.

Laundering procedures in the hospital

A washing machine with good washing action, used with hot water and effective detergents, is essential in the removal of soil and microbial contamination. An accurate thermometer should be used to measure water temperatures. A water temperature above 71°C. (160°F.) for 25 minutes will kill practically all microorganisms except spores. Such a temperature is recommended for use with all except delicate fabrics such as woolens, nylon, and the like. It is easier to disinfect cotton thermal blankets than woolen blankets, because of the reaction of wool to hot water. Laundering delicate fabrics at lower temperatures may even result in an increase in microbial contamination. Sour, bleach, or other chemical treatments may provide further reduction in microbial contamination beyond the effects of hot water. Although recontamination of washed linen may occur during extraction, drying and ironing substantially reduce the levels of microbial contamination of linen.

It is recommended that all heavily soiled launderable items such as mops and step-off mats be washed separately.

There are advantages to treating linen with textile softeners incorporated into the laundering process. Softeners make the linen easier to wash, easier to handle, and softer for the patient; they also reduce linting. There is no evidence that bacteriostatic additives in laundry rinses affect the incidence of nosocomial infection.

Linen for patients such as severely burned patients, who are particularly susceptible to infections, linens for the nursery, and gowns for obstetrical and operating rooms should be sterilized by autoclaving. Sterilization of linen provides two safety factors: the heat destroys microorganisms not removed in the laundering processes, and the wrappings normally placed around goods as a sterilization procedure protect the linen until it is used.

Laundering procedures outside the hospital

These same standards of quality should be maintained when linen is processed outside the hospital facility. Laundry formulations and temperature levels should be the same as described above. Laundry sorting areas should be separate from processing and packing areas. Special controls are needed in the transportation of linen to ensure delivery of contamination-free linen to the hospital and storage areas. Clean linen should be wrapped in impervious bags or similar protection at the processing site and should remain wrapped until it is ready for use.

Storage

Clean linen should be handled as little as possible and should be covered or wrapped before being stored. Storage in enclosed linen carts, which are wheeled to patient areas, helps to minimize handling of linen as well as to protect it against airborne contamination. Shelves of carts or closets where clean linen is stored must be cleaned on a regular schedule.

Disposable sheets, mattress covers, surgical gowns, and diapers are improving in quality and are also becoming less expensive. There is no evidence that these items alter the incidence of nosocomial infection.

The Housekeeping Department

To the extent that nosocomial infections may be a consequence of exposure to contaminated air, dust, furnishings, equipment, and other fomites, effective environmental sanitation is required to lessen such hazards. Frequent and thorough cleaning of hospital interiors is necessary to reduce the numbers of pathogens. Environmental sanitation is not believed to have as its primary purpose a direct antibacterial effect by the cleaning agents themselves; its main purpose is to physically remove microorganisms from the various fomites that might transmit them to patients.

Cleaning procedures and schedules should be reviewed by the infection control committee. Because of the many complexities of hospital housekeeping, the department head must have a sound working knowledge of the manpower needs, the variations in methods and frequency of cleaning for each section of the hospital, and the pertinent chemical and antimicrobial properties of the cleaning agents to be used. All directives as to cleaning procedures and schedules should be in writing, and each member of the housekeeping staff should be trained to follow them. Inservice training programs should be maintained for new personnel as well as for older employees, to introduce them to new techniques and skills.

Cleaning routines

Inasmuch as cleanliness depends directly upon the frequency and thoroughness of cleaning procedures for the total hospital environment, routine schedules should be established for cleaning of walls, floors, windows, window frames and sills, curtains, bedside screens, fixtures, and furniture throughout the hospital, including the cleaning of waste containers and the collection and disposal of wastes. Waste receptacles should have disposable liners so that both the waste and the liner can be incinerated. In certain areas, such as special treatment rooms, operating rooms, kitchens, and laboratories, the fixtures and furnishings are usually cared for by the nursing service, dietary staff, or technicians and specialized methods are used.

The delivery of clean linen and bedding to wards after room cleaning and the collection of soiled linen, with special provisions for the care of linen from infected patients, must be scheduled if this responsibility has been delegated to the housekeeping department. Specifications for the maintenance and care of equipment and materials used by the housekeeping service must be established so as to minimize chances of bacterial exchange or buildup in the hospital environment. Constant supervision of housekeeping activities must be maintained. Collaboration with the infection control committee is necessary for establishing material and equipment standards and for programming housekeeping activities.

General rules

Except for the ceilings, all horizontal surfaces in patient areas should be wet-cleaned or damp-cleaned at least daily. Uncarpeted floors should be wet-cleaned daily; carpeted floors should be vacuumed daily with equipment that does not add to the microbial load in the air.

The floors in corridors and other open areas should be cleaned once daily with a scrubbing solution that is changed frequently. Cleaning can be accomplished with an automatic scrubber-vacuum machine or by wet mopping in combination with a wet-pickup system. Mopping with a dry, treated dust mop is not recommended. Vacuum cleaning of surfaces for removal of dust and dirt is recommended prior to wet cleaning; however, vacuuming should not be substituted for wet cleaning. Dry buffing of floors may increase the microbial count in the air and is not recommended. Moreover, newer synthetic finishes for floors eliminate the need for routine buffing.

In patient treatment areas, bathroom fixtures, handwashing facilities, and service sinks should be thoroughly cleaned at least daily. Appropriate disinfectants can be chosen to prevent accumulation of certain types of bacteria that are known to create a hazard—for example, the use of 1,000 parts per million free chlorine solutions against pseudomonas.

Terminal cleaning of any room that has been occupied by a patient must be thorough. Contaminated linen and drapes should be handled cautiously to prevent dispersal of organisms. All horizontal surfaces should be washed. Walls need not be routinely cleaned, except for spot cleaning of all visibly soiled areas. Fogging with disinfectants is not recommended (see Fogging, page 62). If the patient area involved is part of a multipatient room, terminal cleaning of this area should follow the above recommendations as much as possible. Airing-out periods are not necessary.

The infection control committee may specify more comprehensive terminal cleaning for isolation rooms vacated by patients with certain highly communicable diseases. In terminal cleaning of an isolation room in which fomites may remain infectious, housekeeping personnel should use the same precautions (immunizations, garb, and protective measures) as recommended for the hospital staff while the patient was hospitalized. Whenever possible, central cleaning and disinfection (or sterilization, if required) is preferable to inroom decontamination for patient care supplies and equipment; suitable protective bagging or covering and labeling should be used in sending contaminated objects to central supply.

Cleaning agents and apparatus

The question as to whether a disinfectant should be mixed with a detergent or should be used separately is largely a matter of economics. The main object is to simplify methods as much as possible, while reducing bacterial content. The first criterion in the selection of a general cleaning agent is that it must be effective in the removal of all kinds of dirt. The second criterion relates to the nature of the dirt itself. The tendency of dirt to disseminate bacterial agents is greatest when the dirt is finely divided and dry. The surfactant power of a cleaning agent is most effective against dirt in the form of oily, greasy, or dried protein deposits.

Reliable disinfectants should be used in areas known to be contaminated with pathogenic bacteria, as in those areas where active infection has been treated. Different kinds of disinfectants vary in their reactions to different kinds of bacteria. For example, phenolic compounds are most active against typhoid, dysentery, and other gram-negative bacteria; quaternary ammonium compounds are active only against staphylococci and streptococci; and iodophores (450 parts per million) have a broad spectrum of action, including a strong bactericidal effect on tubercle bacilli. In all cases, however, the potential danger of the compounds used and their toxicities should be clearly known by those who use them. The staff should also be informed as to which materials may weaken or neutralize these compounds. For example, soap or cotton will inactivate quaternary compounds; various metals may interact with iodine; and proteins, with phenols (see Sterilization and Disinfection, page 93).

The cleaning equipment itself must be constructed of noncorrosive materials; carts should be chosen for ease of cleaning. Mopheads and dusters must be of materials that can be laundered daily; otherwise, disposable materials should be used. Mechanical equipment must be chosen and its upkeep planned with the intention of preventing the spread of bacteria. Wet-pickup and dry vacuums must have efficient filters in order to prevent bacteria from passing through in small dust particles or in aerosol droplets; such filters should be changed regularly.

Fogging

Fogging is the process of nebulization of an aerosol of water or an aqueous solution containing detergents and/or disinfectants within a closed space, such as a vacated hospital room. The mist is dispersed by a generator until all surfaces are wet. Antiseptics commonly employed include quaternary ammonium compounds, phenolics, and hypochlorite solutions. Of these, the quaternary ammonium compounds have been used most frequently.

Organisms may be suspended in air as individual organisms or, more commonly, as droplet nuclei. They may remain suspended and viable in air for several hours. Ultimately, even the lighter particles settle out. The fogging action is dependent upon mist, and moisture increases the rate of sedimentation whether the mist contains an antiseptic or not. Although numerous studies have been designed to demonstrate the effect of fogging on decontamination of hospital rooms, numerous variables make interpretation difficult.

The only benefit of fogging is to remove floating infectious particles from the air, so in rooms with windows that can be opened the particles can be cleared by simply opening the windows. In rooms with forced-air ventilation and in isolation rooms meeting the current standards of at least six exchanges per hour of room air, the vast majority of microorganisms are removed within a short period.

Bacteria that remain on the floor and horizontal surfaces must be removed by mechanical cleansing, regardless of whether or not fogging has been used. Even though effective disinfectants are employed in solution in the fogging process, they must come in direct contact with the microorganisms in order to work. Usually these organisms are protected by organic material, such as blood, secretions of various types, or dirt on the various flat surfaces in the hospital room.

Furthermore, air currents generated by fogging do not result in adequate exposure of vertical surfaces, because the airstream is interrupted as the mist approaches vertical surfaces. Actually, walls and ceilings present little hazard to patients, and the obviously contaminated structures must be hand-cleaned as part of the terminal disinfection process, regardless of whether fogging has been used. The failure of fogging to reach corners, closets, and so forth, similarly presents little hazard, because it is unlikely that the organisms found there would be dispersed and present problems for the next occupant of the room.

Although psychological benefits for both staff members and patients have been attributed to the fogging process, it is important to note that the actual effect of the fogging process is no better than the quality of housekeeping procedures used to remove the moisture and cleanse the walls and floor.

In summary, the rapid precipitation of microorganisms and droplet nuclei from air by a mist vapor is of little advantage in a well-ventilated room or one with modern air-circulation devices. Any advantage of fogging may be more than counterbalanced by the potential damage to horizontal and floor surfaces as a result of using detergent-germicide solutions and by the delay in readying rooms for new occupants. Therefore, fogging is not recommended.

The Engineering and Maintenance Departments

A hospital cannot function efficiently without systematic inspection and preventive maintenance of all equipment, established routines for emergency repair, and proper care of its entire physical structure. The maintenance department must establish effective cooperation with the housekeeping and nursing departments, in order to develop a system for prompt notification and repair of defects in both the building and the service equipment. The maintenance department must also develop adequate routines for the inspection and servicing of all plumbing, heating, refrigerating, electrical, and air-conditioning systems. Another maintenance responsibility is the regular checking of all steam supplies and of utility room equipment, such as autoclaves, that depend upon the proper quantity and quality of steam. Special arrangements for checking and servicing of antibacterial air-filtration systems, in cooperation with the infection control committee, is another maintenance task. The department must also establish procedures for the emergency repair of all essential equipment, day and night.

Specific duties

The maintenance department should be charged with the following specific duties. The filters of all air-handling units should be given frequent inspection, cleaning, and replacement. The air-handling systems must provide delivery of proper air current patterns at all times. The heating and cooling systems must provide optimal temperatures and humidities during all seasons. All air-conditioner cooling coils and drip pans need routine maintenance and cleaning to prevent bacterial and slime growth.

The food serving units using refrigeration or hot service elements must be checked for operation at proper temperatures. The food serving and preparation equipment must be kept clean at all times.

All surfaces—floors, walls, and ceilings—require constant inspection and immediate repair when necessary, in order to maintain smooth, dry, and cleanable surfaces. Any openings or breaks in the walls, foundations, window frames, and so on require immediate repair in order to preserve a clean environment.

Vacuum breakers must be installed in water supply lines wherever necessary and must be checked frequently to ensure proper operation. Indirect waste vents (air gaps) must be installed in liquid waste plumbing in accordance with building codes, and must be checked frequently for stoppage. Water traps should be filled at all times. Water supply lines must be disinfected by chlorination following repairs or service disruptions. Overhead waste lines must be inspected frequently for leakage, as must distilled water equipment.

Miscellaneous duties

Maintenance is also responsible for regularly checking blade handle faucets of handwashing facilities for proper functioning. Spray heads, if used, must be removed and cleaned regularly. Faucet aerators should not be used. Refrigerators in kitchens, laboratories, pharmacy, blood bank, and similar locations must be equipped with thermometers; maintenance personnel must check these routinely to ensure that proper temperatures are maintained. Alarm lights or bells should be installed for critical units. The department must routinely clean autoclave chamber drain screens, calibrate sterilizer thermometers, and maintain operative efficiency of recording devices. Maintenance must also check sterilizer valves and regulating equipment to ensure proper operation. Routine cleaning and sterilization of humidification aerosol generators to prevent bacterial growth in air-conditioning equipment is also a maintenance responsibility, as is routine inspection of gaskets and springs on doors of linen and rubbish chutes, to ensure a tight closure. The control of mice, roaches, and other vermin should be carried out by, or supervised by, this department.

In general, maintenance must keep all housekeeping equipment in good repair and in a sanitary condition in order to maintain a desirable environment within the hospital. It is obvious that a planned, active preventive maintenance program, coordinated with an effective housekeeping program, is essential within each hospital as a step in controlling transmissible infection.

BIBLIOGRAPHY

THE PHYSICIAN

Himmelsbach, C. K. The physician's role in hospital infection control. *GP.* 33:103, June 1966.

THE EPIDEMIOLOGIST

Fuerst, H. T., and others. Hospitals and health department cooperate in hospital epidemiology program. *Hospitals, J.A.H.A.* 41:116, Jan. 16, 1967.

THE NURSE

Anderson, L. C., and Himmelsbach, C. K. The nurse: first line of defense against infections. *Hospitals, J.A.H.A.* 41:84, Oct. 1, 1967.

Seedor, M. M. *Introduction to Asepsis, Programmed Unit in Fundamentals of Nursing.* Rev. ed. New York City: Teachers College, Columbia University, 1964.

Seidler, F. M. Adapting nursing procedures for reverse isolation. *Amer. J. Nurs.* 65:108, June 1965.

THE MICROBIOLOGICAL LABORATORY

American Public Health Association. *Diagnostic Procedures and Reagents.* 4th ed. New York City: APHA, 1963.

Bauer, J. D., and others, editors. *Bray's Clinical Laboratory Methods.* 7th ed. St. Louis: C. V. Mosby Co., 1968.

Herman, L. G., and Himmelsbach, C. K. Detection and control of hospital sources of flavobacteria. *Hospitals, J.A.H.A.* 39:72, June 16, 1965.

Mallison, G. F. Introduction to microbiology of the institutional environment. In: *Proceedings of the Fourth Annual Technical Meeting of the American Association for Contamination Control.* 6-1:1, May 1965. Boston: AACC, 1965.

THE PHARMACY

U.S. National Institutes of Health. *Biological Products, Public Health Service Regulations, Title 42, Part 73* (PHS No. 437). Bethesda, Md.: Division of Biologic Standards, National Institutes of Health, 1969.

THE CENTRAL SUPPLY SERVICE

Standard, P. G., and others. Microbial penetration of muslin- and paper-wrapped sterile packs stored on open shelves and in closed cabinets. *Appl. Microbiol.* 22:432, Sept. 1971.

—————————. Microbial penetration through three types of double wrappers for sterile packs. *Appl. Microbiol.* 26:59, July 1973.

U.S. Public Health Service. *A Manual for Hospital Central Medical and Surgical Supply Services* (PHS No. 930-C-13). Washington, D.C.: U.S. Government Printing Office, 1962.

THE FOOD SERVICE DEPARTMENT

American Hospital Association. *Food Service Manual for Health Care Institutions*. Chicago: AHA, 1972.

Reimer, A. O., and Tillotson, J. L. Food service procedures for reverse isolation. *J. Amer. Diet. Assn.* 48:381, May 1966.

Sanders, E., and others. An outbreak of hospital-associated infections due to *Salmonella derby*. *J. Amer. Med. Assn.* 186:984, Dec. 14, 1963.

Stauffer, L. D. Sanitation in hospital food service. *Hospitals, J.A.H.A.* 38:162, July 16, 1964; 80, Aug. 1, 1964; 84, Aug. 16, 1964; 116, Sept. 1, 1964; 88, Sept. 16, 1964.

U.S. Public Health Service. *Food Service Sanitation Manual* (PHS No. 934). Washington, D.C.: U.S. Government Printing Office, 1962.

THE LAUNDRY AND LINEN SERVICE

American Nursing Home Association. *Handling, Selection, and Use of Linens in Nursing Homes and Related Facilities*. Washington, D.C.: ANHA, 1965.

Caplan, H. Observations on the role of hospital blankets as reservoirs of infection. *J. Hyg.* 60:401, Sept. 1962.

Church, E. D. Hospital laundry hazards leading to recontamination of washed bedding. In: *Proceedings of the National Conference on Institutionally Acquired Infections*. Minneapolis, Minn., Sept. 4-6, 1963 (PHS No. 1188). Washington, D.C.: U.S. Government Printing Office, 1964, pp. 70-77.

Lawrence, C. A., and Maffia, A. J. The use of antiseptic impregnation of fabrics in the treatment and prevention of disease. *Bull. Amer. Soc. Hosp. Pharm.* 14:164, Mar.-Apr. 1957.

McNeil, E., and Choper, E. A. Disinfectants in home laundering. *Soap & Chemical Specialties*. 38:51, Aug. 1962.

Meilicke, C. A., and Smith, N. P. Treating linens for patient safety and comfort. *Hospitals, J.A.H.A.* 36:92, Oct. 16, 1962.

Ridenour, G. M. *A Bacteriological Study of Automatic Clothes Washing*. Ann Arbor, Mich.: National Sanitation Foundation, 1952.

Rubbo, S. D. The role of textiles in hospital cross-infection. In: Williams, R. E. O., and Shooter, R. A., editors. *Infection in Hospitals: Epidemiology and Control*. Philadelphia: F. A. Davis Co., 1963, pp. 231-50.

Sandiford, B. R., and others. Sluicing of hospital linens in automatic washing machines. *Monthly Bull. Ministry of Health and Pub. Health Lab. Serv.* 18:110, June 1959.

Sherrill, J. C., and Kinard, C. L. Sterility of laundered fabrics. *J. Amer. Med. Assn.* 159:1478, Dec. 10, 1955.

Wiksell, J. C., and others. Survival of microorganisms in laundered polyester-cotton sheeting. *Appl. Microbiol.* 25:431, Mar. 1973.

Wiley, H. M. Infection-control measures in the hospital laundry. *Hospitals, J.A.H.A.* 35:66, Dec. 16, 1961.

THE HOUSEKEEPING DEPARTMENT

American Hospital Association. *Housekeeping Manual for Health Care Facilities.* Chicago: AHA, 1966.

Gonzaga, A. J., and others. Transmission of staphylococci by fomites. *J. Amer. Med. Assn.* 189:711, Sept. 7, 1964.

Koren, H. Self inspection program raises cleanliness level. *Hospitals, J.A.H.A.* 42:107, Feb. 16, 1968.

Mallison, G. F. Introduction to microbiology of the institutional environment. In: *Proceedings of the Fourth Annual Technical Meeting of the American Association for Contamination Control.* 6-1:1, May 1965. Boston: AACC, 1965.

FOGGING

Davis, R. N. Effect of fogging on microbial contamination. *Hospitals, J.A.H.A.* 42:69, Mar. 1, 1968.

Fogging, an ineffective measure. Center for Disease Control. *National Nosocomial Infections Study Quarterly Report.* Third Quarter 1971, May 1972.

Hall, L. B. Questions and Answers Section. Room sterilization. *J. Amer. Med. Assn.* 181:462, Aug. 4, 1962.

Walter, C. W., and Errera, D. Fogging. O. R. Question Box. *Hosp. Top.* 42:111, Mar. 1964.

Williams, R. E. O., and Shooter, R. A., editors. *Infection in Hospitals: Epidemiology and Control.* A symposium organized by the Council for International Organizations of Medical Sciences, under the joint auspices of UNESCO and WHO. Philadelphia: F. A. Davis Co., 1963, pp. 235-39.

Chapter 5

Prevention and Control of Infection

Among the methods for the prevention and control of infection within the hospital discussed in this chapter are the control of infection hazards in the hospital environment, architectural planning of hospital facilities, reduction of the chances of acquiring infection directly from patients, suppression of the source of infection, and techniques of hand washing. Procedures and suggestions for isolation and antibiotic prophylaxis are included, as well as methods of sterilization and disinfection appropriate to a strong program of infection control.

ARCHITECTURAL CONSIDERATIONS

The general control of infection in hospitals is influenced to a large degree by the techniques used in the routine daily functions of patient care. These techniques, in turn, are affected by the overall excellence and adaptability of the hospital design itself. In short, a good infection control program can operate more effectively if all departments are able to function smoothly in well-designed facilities.

The basic problems in hospital design include traffic patterns; systems for handling materials, equipment, and wastes; ventilation systems and airflow control; ease in cleaning surfaces and materials; and facilities for implementing infection control.

Traffic Patterns

The traffic flow of persons within a hospital is worthy of attention, because people are the major source of pathogenic organisms and the chance of infection increases whenever and wherever people congregate. Although it is impossible to detect every carrier of virulent microorganisms among staff, patients, and visitors, it is possible to limit to some degree certain spheres of unnecessary human contact, and thereby to lessen opportunities for the spreading or receiving of infectious agents by person-to-person transfer.

Design is one of the factors that can effect the separation of traffic between clean and contaminated areas. In a surgery department, for example, a well-considered design for traffic flow can decrease contacts between infected and noninfected patients. The location of surgical areas can be such that every entrant must pass through the dressing and gowning rooms before he enters.

The best design for separation of traffic through clean and contaminated areas is useless, however, if staff members are assigned to concurrent handling of infected and noninfected patients. In obstetrics, surgery, and pediatrics, discrimination between infected and noninfected patients is generally practiced in staff assignments. This policy is desirable for other departments as well.

Materials Handling

A satisfactory design should eliminate opportunities for soiled materials to come into contact with clean ones. For example, separate mechanical conveyors or dumbwaiters should be used for transporting clean supplies into the departments of surgery or obstetrics and for returning soiled materials to central supply. Eliminating the need for carts and personnel as conveyors of materials through two such important areas should greatly reduce the problems of traffic management and associated hazards of microbial spread. Through provision for the handling of sterile supplies, food, laundry, and other materials, well-designed traffic patterns can reduce opportunities for the spread of infectious agents by direct contact.

In areas other than surgery and pediatrics, current practices make it extremely difficult to prevent contacts between clean and soiled materials. With proper bagging, however, both clean and dirty linens could conceivably be transferred through the same conveyor. Separate conveyors would be preferable for the distribution of food and for the return of dirty dishes, because of the difficulties in protecting clean food.

Laundry chutes and trash chutes are particularly convenient as a means for quick disposal of laundry or trash from a hospital floor, but they have disadvantages, especially in relation to fire hazards and decontamination. However, both laundry and trash, if properly bagged or contained, can be transferred satisfactorily by chutes to the laundry or incinerator. Pneumatic chutes may prove effective for the safe handling of these materials, although results of studies of these chutes are as yet inconclusive.

Mechanical conveyors can facilitate efficient distribution of supplies. However, they must be designed so they do not contribute to fire or infection hazards. Safe design usually includes enclosing conveyors in individual shafts, either horizontal or vertical, with terminal portions opening into separate rooms. These terminal rooms help reduce the flue action of conveyor shafts. In the surgical suite, such terminal rooms are much safer than a conveyor that discharges directly into a clean workroom or into a substerilizing room adjacent to an operating room. The ends of some conveyors cannot be closed off by a door because tote-boxes roll automatically out of the shaft as they arrive. If food is distributed by conveyors, the designer must take special care that the conveyor does not form a passage for the flow of air from soiled areas directly to the kitchen. In such cases it is particularly important to control the flue action.

Ventilation Systems

An adequate ventilation system requires proper design and maintenance in order to keep microbial contamination of the environment at a low level. The prevalence of airborne microorganisms, many of which are potentially pathogenic, is beyond question. These microorganisms, attached to dust, lint, respiratory droplets, or other particles, can cause infection by way of uncontrolled air currents. These problems may result from a hospital design that permits airborne contamination in uncontrolled airstreams to go from one area of the hospital to another. This situation may be particularly serious if contaminated air is allowed to infiltrate areas housing susceptible patients or sterile equipment and supplies. Airborne pathogenic microorganisms may settle on an open surgical wound or on sterile equipment and supplies.

Vents and filters

It is generally accepted that fresh air, properly filtered and tempered, is the ideal medium for the dilution and removal of bacterial and odorous airborne contamination. Desirable ventilation rates, expressed in air changes per hour, vary in accordance with the functions performed in a particular area. It is agreed, however, that the sensitive areas of a hospital—notably the operating rooms, delivery rooms, and nurseries—should be provided with air as nearly bacteria-free as possible.

Certain principles of air circulation must be observed in order to accomplish this objective. For example, all outdoor air inlets should be located as high as possible above ground level; inlets should be remote from ventilation discharge outlets, incinerators, or boiler stacks.

Filters used in the ventilation systems should be selected with particular reference to the functions to be carried out in the area where they are installed. High-efficiency filters should be provided in systems serving areas where patients are particularly susceptible to infection or where certain clinical procedures may subject patients to unusual hazard.

The location of air inlets and exhaust outlets in a room influences the movement of air within the area. High wall or ceiling inlets and low wall outlets are recommended for all sensitive areas. These locations are also highly desirable for vents in areas subject to heavy contamination, such as necropsy rooms, isolation rooms, and treatment rooms. Such locations move the clean air downward through the occupied area toward the contaminated floor area, where it is removed at the low exhaust outlets.

A system of regular inspection and maintenance of the filters, humidifiers, and grilles in the air supply system is important in preventing the development of reservoirs of organisms.

Zoning

Departmental zoning of air systems helps to confine the air of a department to that department alone. It also reduces the probability that air from a particular clinical unit will become mixed with that from another unit or with air from the dietary or administrative areas.

A design that enables air pressure to control air movement into or out of a specific room or area is effective in controlling the spread of contamination. Effective air pressurization is impossible without keeping all doors closed except for necessary entrances and exits.

Positive air pressure is recommended for sensitive areas. Such pressure is obtained by supplying more ventilating air into an area than can be removed from it by the exhaust ventilation system. This induced pressurization produces an outflow around doors and other openings, and lessens infiltration of air from more contaminated areas.

Negative air pressure, which is recommended for contaminated areas, can be obtained by supplying less air to the area than can be removed by the ventilation system. Negative air pressure produces an inflow around openings and reduces the possibility of contaminated air leaving the area.

Unidirectional (Laminar) Clean Airflow

A unidirectional clean airflow system admits air into a room through one entire side and allows it to escape through multiple large openings on the opposite side. Without such a laminar flow system, even with modern conventional ventilation and air-conditioning systems, air currents move freely in all directions when air is forced through and emerges from small ducts. Air that is deflected by whatever objects may obstruct it is said to be flowing in a turbulent manner. Turbulence facilitates dispersal of viable pathogenic bacteria that may be contained in small dust particles or droplet nuclei. Such particles are usually more than four microns in diameter.

The air in a unidirectional system should travel at a velocity of at least 100 feet per minute. Unobstructed air currents travel through the room in straight lines and do not deviate or become turbulent. Transient turbulence may occur if the airflow is deflected by an obstacle, but the flow quickly resumes its uniform pattern after the obstacle has been removed or the air progresses farther to its point of egress from the room. By avoiding turbulence, droplet nuclei and other particles do not accumulate on irregular surfaces but are carried out with the airstream.

For optimal cleanliness, air should be circulated into the room through a high-efficiency particulate air (HEPA) filter, which excludes particulate matter of defined size. If particles 0.3 micron in diameter and larger are removed, the air entering the room will be essentially clean and free of virtually all bacterial contaminants.

In the health fields the principle of laminar flow has been applied to the microbiology laboratory, the pharmacy, special intensive care units, and particularly the operating rooms.

In the microbiology laboratory special unidirectional airflow hoods serve as areas for handling and transferring microbial cultures. These are particularly useful for certain highly infectious cultures. Hoods of this type protect the individual worker as well as the laboratory environment from contamination by the airborne route.

In the pharmacy (see page 49), similar hoods are used to prevent airborne contamination of sterile fluids when containers are opened, for example, when an antibiotic is added to a container of sterile glucose solution for intravenous use or when fluids for parenteral hyperalimentation are prepared.

Portable laminar flow units are available that fit over a hospital bed. The value of these units in reducing the hazard of airborne infection to patients with extensive burns is under investigation.

Because airborne bacteria in the operating room may enter surgical wounds, a possible source of infection might be reduced if the air entering the room were sterile. Operations involving prosthetic devices, such as total replacement of the hip, have resulted in greater attention to asepsis. These prostheses are foreign bodies, favoring persistence of sepsis should infection occur at the time of surgery. Other sources of infection are bacteria carried by the patient himself, instruments and equipment, and bacteria shed by operating room personnel.

The construction of operating rooms providing filtered unidirectional airflow is an expensive investment. The units and the permanent room-within-a-room glass enclosure commonly referred to as the "greenhouse" are not as adaptable as the present operating rooms for the wide variety of surgical procedures, and thus increase the expense of the units.

There is clear evidence that operating rooms modified or constructed to include appropriate air filters and unidirectional flow devices have lower bacterial counts in the air than rooms not so modified. The limited evidence at this time does not indicate that laminar, clean airflow, in itself, has a favorable influence on the incidence of surgical wound infections. All presently accepted surgical, technical, and hygienic methods of achieving surgical asepsis must be rigidly maintained regardless of the type of air system employed.

Finish Materials

Much is expected from the finish materials used in a hospital. No material presently available, however, seems to have all the desirable characteristics: noise-reducing properties, pleasing appearance, durability, ease in being cleaned, and fire resistance.

The selection of suitable finish materials is difficult. Ease of cleaning is of prime importance in maintaining a clean environment. Durability is also important, because a material that quickly wears, cracks, or deteriorates will also lose its cleaning and esthetic qualities. Ceiling, wall, and floor coverings that are made of squares or tiles have joints, which may be difficult to clean. It is doubtful, however, that such materials are objectionable from the standpoint of ordinary cleanliness.

Acoustical surfaces for walls or ceilings are not satisfactory in areas such as surgery, kitchens, and treatment rooms, where cleaning problems are most important.

Walls and wainscots must be able to withstand considerable wear and impact; they must also have a good appearance and a reasonable cost. Such features are especially important in patients' rooms and in corridors.

Ceramic tile materials provide long-term durability and pleasing appearance in corridors. Floors must be easily cleaned and maintained, as well as be durable in order to take heavy traffic. Most vinyl and vinyl asbestos materials make good floor coverings, because of their durability, resilience, and ease of cleaning.

Carpets

There has been increasing interest in recent years in carpeting of patient care areas of hospitals. Advantages cited for carpets include less maintenance time required than for hard-surfaced floors, reduction of sound levels, lower rates of injury among patients who fall to the floor, and provision of a setting for patients that is warmer and less "institutional." Disadvantages that have been reported for carpets include greater combined cost for installation, maintenance, and replacement than for hard-surfaced floors; increased effort required to move wheeled equipment; production of static electricity; possible fire and smoke hazards; difficulty in removing stains made by food or other spilled materials; and increased maintenance costs due to repair of burns and mechanical injury to the textiles.

Studies of hospital carpeting have been conducted that purport to include valid evaluations of risk of infection associated with carpeted versus hard-surfaced floors. These studies are mainly microbiological evaluations showing that carpets may contain microbial contamination at levels about four orders of magnitude greater per unit area than levels present on hard-surfaced floors. No adequately controlled study of the possible influence of carpets on nosocomial infections has ever been reported; there is no evidence at this time that hospital carpeting is associated with either increased or decreased risk of nosocomial infection as compared with hard-surfaced floors. Despite the lack of clear evidence to the contrary, the potential disadvantage of carpeting is its greater microbial content.

If carpets are used, the following points may be helpful. Carpets installed in institutions must meet the flame-spread requirements of the Health Care Facilities Services, Public Health Service, U.S. Department of Health, Education, and Welfare. Cleaning procedures for acceptable visual appearance must be planned, with consideration given to the expense and time required. Carpets without resilient backing or padding glued directly onto floors provide good appearance and high levels of sound attenuation. These offer less resistance for moving wheeled equipment than fully padded carpets. Pads may increase smoke and fire hazards and create odor problems associated with microbial growth if they become wet. Short-looped pile carpets are easier to clean and are more resistant to staining than higher looped or cut-pile carpets. Carpets with loops of several colors interspersed, rather than solid color carpets, are more likely to maintain good esthetic appearance.

Carpets in areas where traffic is heavy and spillage of liquids on the floor is likely should be the indoor-outdoor type, which can be removed for cleaning. Prompt cleaning of liquid spills on carpets is essential, and thorough daily vacuuming is required to maintain their appearance. Efforts should be made to reduce static electricity in carpets by special treatment and maintenance of relative humidities above 30 per cent. Use of carpets with conductive threads interwoven to ground static charges is required in areas where flammable materials are in use.

Handwashing Facilities

Handwashing facilities should be readily available in all areas of the hospital. For the handwashing lavatory in the patient's room it is generally preferable to have the short lever type of faucet handle. This type of handle is convenient to use; it also is cheaper to install and maintain than are the types designed to avoid use by the hands. For the surgical or obstetrical patient's room and the intensive care unit, elbow-, knee-, or foot-operated controls may be used. There is some question as to whether or not there should be a lavatory in the patient's room when there is an adjacent toilet. Ideally, there should be a lavatory in the toilet room as well as in the patient's room, particularly in multipatient rooms, but this is not always economically feasible. A paper towel dispenser should be located adjacent to every handwashing facility.

General Control

In relation to problems of isolation, aspects of design that should be emphasized are the need for: (1) sufficient space around the bed to carry out all necessary isolation techniques; (2) handwashing facilities, a wall-hung toilet, and a shower; and (3) an anteroom with a lavatory, with closets for clean gowns and other materials, and with space for a container for soiled materials. This anteroom facilitates implementation of isolation techniques without the necessity of using the public corridor. Figure 5, opposite page, shows an isolation room floor plan that includes an anteroom.

Although it is desirable and occasionally necessary—for example, in surgery or in preparation rooms—to separate clean and dirty areas, there are many hospital situations in which soiled materials are introduced into an

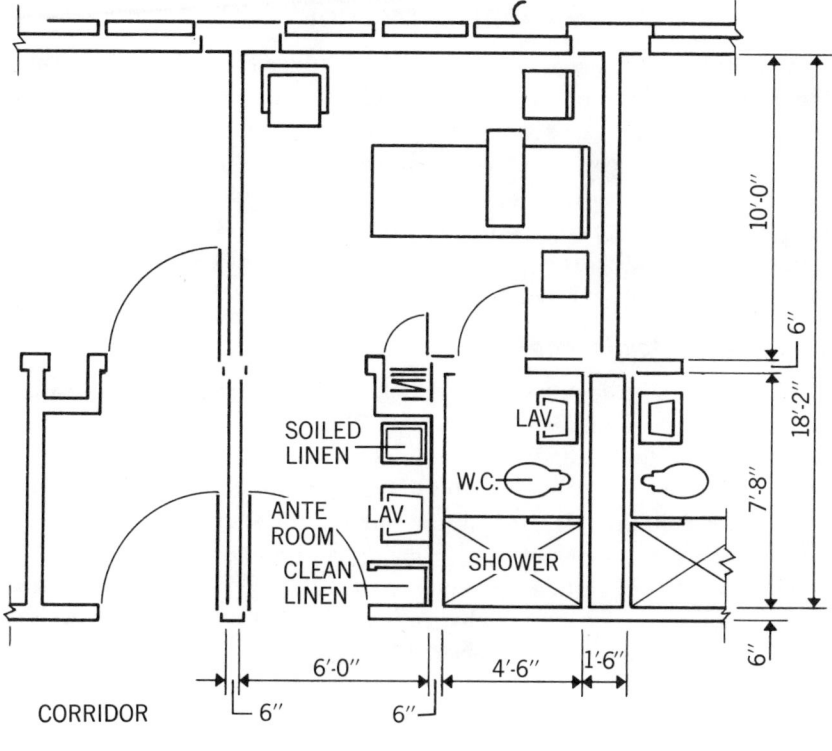

Figure 5
FLOOR PLAN FOR ISOLATION ROOM
Source: U.S. Public Health Service, Division of Hospital and Medical Facilities, Architectural Engineering and Equipment Branch.

area also used for cleaning, sterilizing, or storing. This situation may occur in floor utility rooms, anesthesiologists' workrooms, and similar areas. In such cases, strict techniques and careful supervision must be practiced to avoid accidental contamination of clean materials, especially in the cleanup room of central supply or the sorting room and wash room of the laundry. A pass-through sterilizer can be useful in such situations, as the sterilizer is loaded on the soiled side and the materials are discharged into the clean work area. In laundries, a double-door washing machine and extractor can be helpful. These types of equipment allow simple techniques and require little supervision, because the physical arrangement of space and equipment precludes accidental contact between dirty and clean materials.

ENVIRONMENTAL CONTROL

Although most exogenous nosocomial infections result from direct personal contact, some result from contamination of the physical environment. For example, it is well established that certain infectious agents, such as staphylococci, streptococci, and tubercle bacilli, can survive for various periods on surfaces or in dust. This environmental contamination can be reduced or prevented by careful attention to cleanliness and sanitation. Appropriate preventive measures are discussed under the headings of airborne and surface contamination.

Airborne Contamination

An outline of sources, types of organisms, and control measures relating to airborne contamination is shown in Table 7, below. Infection from droplet nuclei, for example, can be minimized through education in personal hygiene. Face masks are useful in the operating room or for personnel in, but not regularly assigned to, the nursery. However, masks lose their effectiveness with time, moisture, or handling during use.

The potential of certain personnel to shed staphylococci from skin surfaces is not apparent from a physical examination of the patient or the employee. Although often associated with chronic dermatitis, shedding

Table 7

AIRBORNE CONTAMINATION CONTROL

Sources	Type of organisms	Control measures
Droplet nuclei* from the respiratory tract of personnel, patients, and visitors	Pneumococci Respiratory viruses Streptococci Staphylococci Tubercle bacilli	Exclusion of staff when ill; staff training and education in personal hygiene; masks in special cases
Organisms shed from the skin during activity	Staphylococci	Exclusion of staff with furuncles or similar lesions
Routine patient care procedures	Staphylococci and others	Care in bedmaking and sweeping; medical asepsis; decontamination of equipment after each use
Aerosol droplets from ventilating equipment, humidifiers, basins, and sinks	Pseudomonas and other gram-negative	Proper maintenance, use of neoprene gaskets
Dust from animal rooms	Various gram-negative	Proper location and ventilation

*All except tuberculosis are droplet-spread infections and thus not truly airborne.

may occur with normal skin. Removal of hospital employees from patient care responsibilities is not warranted on the basis of skin cultures alone, since neither Rodac plate samples nor swabs give reliable information as to the numbers of pathogenic organisms actually shed. However, epidemiologic evidence of the subject's association with clinical illness should be used as a realistic indication of hazard.

Microorganisms on the floor or other surfaces may become airborne during certain routine patient care procedures. The problem is of particular importance in hospitals with less than optimal ventilation. Practices particularly likely to produce airborne contamination include sweeping, using dry dust mops or dry dust cloths, using mechanical buffers and unfiltered vacuum cleaners, shaking linen when changing beds, and using laundry chutes that do not have self-closing doors. Dusty or potentially infectious wastes originating in the patient room can be satisfactorily handled in waxed or plastic waste bags. Use of such bags not only avoids air contamination when wastes are emptied but also minimizes problems associated with contaminated wastebaskets.

Ventilating and air-conditioning equipment may serve as sources of airborne contamination, particularly if moisture from condensation or sprayed coils is present without adequate downstream air filtration.

Animals kept for laboratory use may be a source of airborne contamination, frequently of the gram-negative variety. Measures for controlling this type of airborne contamination should begin with situating animal rooms in the service area of the hospital and under negative air pressure with respect to patient care areas. Keeping exhaust air filters clean and providing relatively high ventilation rates—10 to 15 air changes per hour—are also effective infection control measures. The use of dustless animal bedding is important in maintaining a high level of general cleanliness. Ventilated cages or negative pressure plastic isolators can be used if the problem is severe.

Surface Contamination

Most airborne and surface contamination eventually descends to floors. Because shoes or wheels pick up microorganisms from floors and spread them from room to room, floors are among the most highly microbially contaminated areas of a hospital. Even though routine bacteriological samples taken from floors are used by some hospitals as gross indicators of such contamination, such sampling programs are not recommended, inasmuch as there are no accepted standards of microbiological cleanliness of floors.

Although it has been demonstrated that total bacterial counts after cleaning with a good soap or detergent alone are as low as after cleaning with a disinfectant, there are strong arguments in favor of using a disinfectant chosen for its ability to kill particular pathogens known to be present in wards and special treatment areas. Commercial formulations most commonly contain a phenolic (a chlorophenol) in order to get efficient action against gram-negative organisms yet still kill staphylococci reasonably well.

Frequent changes of cleaning solutions and daily laundering and thorough drying of mops are recommended. Painted walls, with smooth surfaces that are easily washed, rarely present a contamination problem.

Other Contamination

General considerations should result in a minimal amount of available food for insects and rodents. With regard to rodent control, use of poisoned bait has disadvantages. Use of traps, though more expensive in terms of manpower, is usually preferable for hospitals. Placing traps in animal rooms at a density of about one or two traps per 100 square feet usually controls escaped laboratory rodents. Traps may be set elsewhere when a specific problem exists. With regard to insect control, areas other than patient care areas can be treated routinely with either pyrethrum or residual insecticides, if adequate precautions are taken. In patient rooms, it is generally preferable to use insecticides for a definite and specific problem only. Whether patients should be removed while the insecticide is being used depends on the type of insecticide, the extent of the procedure, and the condition of the patient. Insecticides having the lowest toxicity level for humans should be used.

ISOLATION TECHNIQUES AND PROCEDURES

The best means available to prevent the spread of infection from a patient to other patients, personnel, visitors, and the environment is to establish an aseptic barrier around the patient. Such containment of the offending microorganisms is commonly called isolation but is also referred to as barrier nursing. Because the practice of isolation is difficult and time consuming, it is important that it be specifically suited to both the patient and the disease to be controlled and that its practice be limited to procedures of demonstrated value.

The infection control committee should develop and recommend isolation policies and procedures, and these should be implemented by the administration. The committee should review procedures from time to time and modify policies and methods as necessary. The infection control nurse should be knowledgeable in and should serve as the consultant on methods of isolation.

Routes of Spread

The requirements for isolation vary according to the route by which the disease is spread. There are two main transmission routes for which isolation techniques are invoked: contact and airborne. The contact route includes some respiratory and enteric agents as well as agents associated with infections of the skin. Some agents are spread by both routes. Examples of the different routes are indicated in Table 2, page 8.

Diseases with mixed modes of spread should be treated under a more comprehensive form of isolation. Because of high virulence and great communicability, strict isolation is recommended for diphtheria, eczema vaccinatum, neonatal vesicular disease (herpes simplex), congenital rubella, smallpox, and staphylococcal and streptococcal pneumonia. Diseases requiring only respiratory isolation are chickenpox, herpes zoster (pediatrics), measles, meningococcal infections, mumps, pertussis, rubella, and pulmonary tuberculosis. Enteric isolation should be used for diseases such as cholera, enteropathogenic *Escherichia coli* gastroenteritis, hepatitis A or B, salmonellosis, and shigellosis. Wound and skin isolation should be used for skin infections, burns, gas gangrene, and impetigo.

Specific Requirements

Ordinarily, isolation should be ordered by the attending physician. As a safeguard, however, it is recommended that the hospital establish a standing order that permits a charge nurse to put an infected patient in isolation for up to 48 hours if a physician is not available to make the determination. The charge nurse should report this action to both the attending physician and the infection control officer as soon as possible.

Protective measures. Isolation requirements vary with the nature of infection, condition and behavior of the patient, and facilities available. Figures 6 through 10, pages 82-86, demonstrate the card system developed by the Public Health Service to give concise information about isolation procedures for specific communicable diseases.*

---

*Figures 6 through 10 are adapted from U.S. Public Health Service Publication No. 2054. Each self-adhesive card can be ordered individually or in sets of 100. Order from the Superintendent of Documents, U.S. Government Printing Office, Washington, D.C. 20402. The cards can also be prepared by an individual hospital according to its needs.

Enteric Precautions
Visitors—Report to Nurses' Station Before Entering Room

1. **Private Room**—*necessary for children only.*
2. **Gowns**—must be worn by all persons having direct contact with patient.
3. **Masks**—not necessary.
4. **Hands**—must be washed on entering and leaving room.
5. **Gloves**—must be worn by all persons having direct contact with patient or with articles contaminated with fecal material.
6. **Articles**—special precautions necessary for articles contaminated with urine and feces. Articles must be disinfected or discarded.

Front

Diseases Requiring Enteric Precautions*

1. **Cholera**
2. **Diarrhea—acute illness with suspected infectious etiology**
3. **Enterocolitis, staphylococcal**
4. **Gastroenteritis caused by**
   a. Enterotoxic (enteropathogenic) *Escherichia coli*
   b. Salmonella species
   c. Shigella species
   d. *Yersinia enterocolitica*
5. **Hepatitis, viral Type A or Type B**
6. **Typhoid fever**

*See *Isolation Techniques for Use in Hospitals* for details and recommended duration of isolation.

PHS Publication No. 2054-D

Back

Figure 6
CARD DESCRIBING ENTERIC PRECAUTIONS

Protective Isolation

Visitors—Report to Nurses' Station Before Entering Room

1. **Private Room**—*necessary;* door must be kept closed.
2. **Gowns**—must be worn by all persons entering room.
3. **Masks**—must be worn by all persons entering room.
4. **Hands**—must be washed on entering and leaving room.
5. **Gloves**—must be worn by all persons having direct contact with patient.
6. **Articles**—see *Isolation Techniques for Use in Hospitals*.

Front

Conditions That May Require Protective Isolation*

1. Agranulocytosis
2. Certain patients with extensive noninfected burns
3. Dermatitis—noninfected vesicular, bullous, or eczematous disease when severe and extensive
4. Certain patients receiving immunosuppressive therapy
5. Certain patients with lymphomas and leukemia

*See *Isolation Techniques for Use in Hospitals* for details and recommended duration of isolation.

PHS Publication No. 2054-C

Back

Figure 7
CARD DESCRIBING PROTECTIVE ISOLATION

Respiratory Isolation

Visitors—Report to Nurses' Station Before Entering Room

1. **Private Room**—*necessary;* door must be kept closed.
2. **Gowns**—not necessary.
3. **Masks**—must be worn unless person entering room is not susceptible to the disease.
4. **Hands**—must be washed on entering and leaving room.
5. **Gloves**—not necessary.
6. **Articles**—those contaminated with secretions must be disinfected.

Front

Diseases Requiring Respiratory Isolation*

1. Measles (rubeola)
2. Meningitis, meningococcal
3. Meningococcemia
4. Mumps
5. Pertussis (whooping cough)
6. Rubella (German measles), except congenital rubella syndrome
7. Tuberculosis, pulmonary—sputum positive or suspect

*See *Isolation Techniques for Use in Hospitals* for details and recommended duration of isolation.

PHS Publication No. 2054-B

Back

Figure 8
CARD DESCRIBING RESPIRATORY ISOLATION

Strict Isolation

Visitors—Report to Nurses' Station Before Entering Room

1. **Private Room**—*necessary;* door must be kept closed.
2. **Gowns**—must be worn by all persons entering room.
3. **Masks**—must be worn by all persons entering room.
4. **Hands**—must be washed on entering and leaving room.
5. **Gloves**—must be worn by all persons entering room.
6. **Articles**—must be discarded, or wrapped before being sent to Central Supply for disinfection or sterilization.

Front

Diseases Requiring Strict Isolation*

1. Anthrax, inhalation
2. Burn wound, extensive, infected with
   a. *Staphylococcus aureus,* or
   b. Group A streptococcus
3. Congenital rubella syndrome
4. Diphtheria
5. Disseminated neonatal *Herpesvirus hominis* (herpes simplex)
6. Plague, pulmonic
7. Pneumonia, infected with
   a. *Staphylococcus aureus,* or
   b. Group A streptococcus
8. Rabies
9. Skin infection, extensive, with
   a. *Staphylococcus aureus,* or
   b. Group A streptococcus
10. Smallpox
11. Vaccinia
    a. Generalized and progressive
    b. Eczema vaccinatum
12. Varicella and disseminated herpes zoster

*See *Isolation Techniques for Use in Hospitals* for details and recommended duration of isolation.

PHS Publication No. 2054-A

Back

Figure 9
CARD DESCRIBING STRICT ISOLATION

Wound & Skin Precautions
Visitors—Report to Nurses' Station Before Entering Room

1. **Private Room**—desirable.
2. **Gowns**—must be worn by all persons having direct contact with patient.
3. **Masks**—not necessary except during dressing changes.
4. **Hands**—must be washed on entering and leaving room.
5. **Gloves**—must be worn by all persons having direct contact with infected area.
6. **Articles**—special precautions necessary for instruments, dressings, and linen.

NOTE: See *Isolation Techniques for Use in Hospitals* for Special Dressing Techniques to be used when changing dressings.

Front

Diseases Requiring Wound & Skin Precautions*

1. Burns with excessive purulent drainage except those with
    a. *Staphylococcus aureus,* or
    b. Group A streptococcus
2. Gas gangrene
3. Herpes zoster
4. Melioidosis
5. Plague, bubonic
6. Skin infection, extensive, that cannot be covered by a dressing except those infected with
    a. *Staphylococcus aureus,* or
    b. Group A streptococcus
7. Wound infection with excessive purulent drainage that cannot be covered by a dressing

*See *Isolation Techniques for Use in Hospitals* for details and recommended duration of isolation.

PHS Publication No. 2054-E

Back

Figure 10
CARD DESCRIBING WOUND AND SKIN PRECAUTIONS

For strict and respiratory isolation, the patient should be confined by himself in a room with private toilet, bath, and lavatory; the door to the room should be kept closed under most circumstances.

The specific isolation procedures to be followed should be posted on the door or at the entrance to the room on a chart. The physician or nurse or both should instruct the patient on the reasons for isolation and his participation in it.

Specific precautions to be taken should be ordered by the attending physician in accordance with hospital policy; precautions are applicable to all persons who must deal with the patient. The following measures are recommended:

- Mask: The purpose of a mask is to protect the wearer against acquiring a disease spread by droplets or aerosols. Although wearing a mask does not provide absolute protection to the wearer, a double-thickness, ample-size gauze mask worn well across the nose and mouth is of some help. A clean, fresh mask should be worn each time use of a mask is indicated, and masks should be changed periodically when prolonged single use is required.
- Gown: If the disease for which isolation is prescribed can be transmitted via clothing, a clean gown should be worn by those persons whose duties require contact with the patient or his fomites. A fresh gown should be used on each occasion, and the wearer should dispose of it in an aseptic fashion into a suitable receptacle inside the door prior to leaving the room.
- Hand washing: Staff members in contact with the patient should wash their hands on each occasion before entering and after leaving the isolation room.
- Gloves: When indicated, gloves should be worn for manual contact with the patient, his fomites, or biological materials. The wearer should discard the gloves aseptically into a suitable container prior to leaving the room.

Equipment and supplies. The needs for equipment used in the care of the patient should be anticipated, and such equipment should be assigned to the room for the duration of the isolation. The isolation room should be made as self-sufficient as possible in terms of supplies and equipment. After equipment has been used, it should be cleaned with a detergent and disinfected with a suitable agent.

Sanitation. Daily wet mopping of the floor and other horizontal surfaces with a fresh solution of a suitable germicidal detergent is important. Terminal cleaning should be done in accordance with special procedures approved by the infection control committee and the principles recommended in The Housekeeping Department, page 59. Waste should be collected in a receptacle lined with either a plastic or wax paper bag. The mouth of the bag should be tied securely prior to its removal from the room, and the bag and its contents should be incinerated. Soiled linen should be collected in a color-coded bag within the room. On being taken out of the room, the bag and its contents should be placed in a second color-coded bag prior to its removal to the laundry. Disposable plates and utensils may be used for the isolation patient. If regular hospital dishes and utensils are used, they should be washed last. In either case, the dirty dishes should be removed from the room in a plastic or wax paper bag. As a further measure of protection, the flow of air should move from the corridor through the room to the outside. This can be achieved by having the air pressure lower in the room than that in the corridor, as noted in Ventilation Systems, page 71.

Visitors. Ideally, there should be no visitors in isolation rooms. But the psychological effects of isolation on a patient are of sufficient importance that in most instances some visiting has to be allowed. It is recommended that visiting be permitted only on order of the physician. The nurse should carefully instruct all visitors in asepsis and self-protection; they should wear masks and gowns if necessary; they should have no direct contact with the patient. The visit should be supervised by the nurse, with visiting restricted to no more than two or three adults for one brief period (see Regulations for Hospital Visitors, page 34).

Protective Isolation

Protective isolation is also called reverse isolation. Its purpose is to protect patients with decreased resistance to infection. Reverse isolation does not protect against infection by the patient's endogenous organisms, but it lessens the chances of acquiring infections from others with whom the patient may come into contact. Protective isolation may be recommended for patients with burns; premature infants; patients with profound granulocytopenia; patients with hypo- or agammaglobulinemia; and patients receiving immunosuppressive therapy, prolonged use of antilymphocyte serum, intensive radiation or corticosteroid therapy, such as transplant recipients or those with leukemia or lymphoma.

Reverse isolation as protective management can be successful only through the most scrupulous attention to details. The objective is to maintain the patient at a level of asepsis comparable to that in the operating room. Any source of contamination is potentially dangerous to the patient.

This type of protective isolation is a continuous, 24-hour, day-by-day responsibility.

In the practice of protective isolation, the patient should be assigned to a cleaned, single room with bath and lavatory. Where available, a room provided with ventilation by filtered air under positive pressure is desirable. The patient and his family must be informed of the reasons for the isolation, and all must be given instruction in the fundamental principles of personal hygiene. As in regular isolation procedure, a notice should be placed on the door explaining the measures being taken in this room. The door should always be kept closed except for essential entries and exits, and all persons with definite or suspected infection should be excluded from entering. Attending personnel should enter the room only when necessary, and all personnel and medically authorized visitors should wear clean caps and sterile masks and gowns while in the room. Attending personnel should wear sterile or disposable gloves when it is necessary to touch the patient or to handle objects that are about to come into contact with the patient. Suitable precautions should be taken to make certain that everything that touches the patient is either clean or sterile.

For the patient who is maintained in a plastic isolator or unidirectional (laminar) airflow room, these precautions do not apply, with the exception of the exclusion of all persons with definite or suspected infections.

The need for continued isolation should be reviewed daily.

Simplified Isolation Procedures

The isolation procedures and facilities necessary to implement them, as described previously, represent the ideal situation. Accordingly, compromises must be made in the individual hospital when limitations are imposed by less than ideal physical facilities and by varying patient loads. For example, isolating patients in single rooms may quickly exhaust a hospital's supply of single rooms. Under such circumstances, it is reasonable to isolate two patients with the same disease, such as measles or hepatitis A, in the same two-bed room.

Because of restrictions on the number of available beds, there may be insufficient individual single rooms for isolation purposes. Therefore, some kind of priority ranking for isolation cases should be established and applied. It is more important, for example, to isolate a recalcitrant patient with open pulmonary tuberculosis than a cooperative patient with hepatitis A. Among patients with infections transferred by the enteric route (except for typhoid fever), it is generally more important to isolate those with severe diarrhea than those without.

No hard and fast rules can be stated, but in general the priority of isolation should vary directly with the potential severity of the disease and with the risk of transmission to other patients and to hospital personnel.

Other compromises may become necessary because of the restrictions imposed by the physical design of the hospital. Such modifications must be carefully considered and must be tailored to meet the hospital's needs and to adapt to the hospital's facilities. It is even possible to isolate a patient in an open ward. This involves the use of portable screens, handwashing and rinsing basins, a supply of fresh gowns and masks, and containers for their disposal. Isolation techniques carried out in this fashion are obviously not as complete as those done in a private room, but are certainly preferable to making no attempt whatever to isolate a patient who needs such treatment.

The utilization of an entire ward, wing, or area of a hospital for isolation patients has been adopted by some hospitals. One significant advantage of this technique is that all the nurses working in these areas may be specially trained and experienced in using isolation techniques. The principal disadvantage is the rather wide fluctuation in the number of patients requiring isolation in a hospital from day to day; at times many beds in an isolation facility may be unoccupied. The decision to adopt such a technique must be made by the individual hospital on the basis of the availability of facilities and nursing staff and a realistic estimate of the demand for isolation procedures.

Intensive care units should not be used for isolation. The use of intensive care units has helped in achieving significant improvement in hospital care of many seriously ill patients, as well as more efficient use of nursing personnel. On the other hand, intensive care units are also ideal locations for cross infection when infected patients are permitted in these units. Infected patients and patients requiring isolation techniques should not be permitted in intensive care units unless special arrangements are made to achieve effective isolation (see Hazardous Areas, page 124).

The cost of isolating patients, measured in both time and money, is substantial. This cost is often added directly to the patient's bill. Some hospitals, quite properly, have questioned whether the patient himself should be held liable for the added cost of isolation, particularly if the infection for which he was isolated was acquired in the hospital. It seems much more equitable, considering who is protected by isolating patients, to make no specific charges for isolation as such, but rather to spread the cost among all patients, because they all benefit by the isolation of patients with communicable disease.

ANTIBIOTIC PROPHYLAXIS

Antimicrobial drugs alone do not prevent all types of infection. Some of these drugs can be effective in preventing infection after known exposure to certain specific microorganisms, provided that those organisms are sensitive and accessible to the prophylactic agent. However, antibiotics as ordinarily prescribed are usually not effective in the prophylaxis of such diseases as postoperative wound infection, urinary tract infection, or pneumonia. The use of antibiotics prophylactically tends to promote colonization of contaminated areas and infection with organisms that are resistant to these agents.

Antibiotics comprise a large part of the medications used in hospitals. Unfortunately, and partly because of this fact, microorgansims resistant to antimicrobial drugs are now commonly found in hospitals. These resistant microorganisms are responsible for a substantial portion of nosocomial infections. Consequently, to reduce the emergence of resistant organisms, some hospitals are attempting to restrict the use of all or at least some antimicrobial drugs. The hospital staff should be encouraged to support this practice.

Though the prophylactic use of antimicrobial drugs generally should be restricted, selective prophylactic use of antibiotics may be indicated in the following situations.

Bacterial endocarditis

As a preventive measure against bacterial endocarditis, patients with rheumatic heart disease and some forms of congenital heart disease should be given prophylactic antimicrobial treatment prior to surgery, including oral surgery. A combination of procaine penicillin (IM) and crystalline penicillin, given in appropriate dosage immediately prior to dental manipulation and extraction and on each of the following two days, is one method in current use. In penicillin-sensitive patients, therapeutic doses of clindamycin, erythromycin, or tetracycline can be used instead. Before and after general surgery and genitourinary instrumentations, appropriate dosage of penicillin combined with streptomycin has been considered effective. The infections that occur after the use of prophylactic antibiotics are generally resistant to those antibiotics. Parenteral or oral treatment with penicillinase-resistant penicillins should precede incision and drainage of extensive cutaneous staphylococcal infection.

Gonorrhea

Prophylactic treatment to hospital employees exposed to patients with gonorrhea should not be necessary. Employees should handle contaminated materials with caution. When genital examinations are made, gloves should be worn by the examiner. Upon contamination of the conjunctivae or upon other gross breaks in technique, gonococcal infection can usually be prevented by the administration of penicillin (oral) or procaine penicillin (IM). Erythromycin or tetracycline can be used in persons allergic to penicillin. For the treatment of newborn infants, see Newborn Nursery, page 135.

Group A streptococcal infection

Although aseptic precautions, including protective isolation, constitute the preferred methods, streptococcal infection of wounds and burns can be prevented by the administration of penicillin, or of other antibiotic drugs in penicillin-sensitive persons. Prophylaxis by the use of penicillin has also been effective in preventing colonization and infections with hemolytic streptococcal infections, thereby reducing later complications such as the recurrence of rheumatic fever in susceptible individuals or the glomerulonephritis that follows infections with nephritogenic strains. Hospitalized patients and personnel with a history of rheumatic heart disease or rheumatic fever should receive such prophylactic treatment as recommended by the American Heart Association.

Meningococcal infection

The spread of meningococcal disease in hospitals is rare, though asymptomatic carriers of meningococci may be prevalent among both patients and personnel. For these reasons, prophylactic treatment of hospital personnel exposed to patients with meningococcal infection is not necessary except under unusual circumstances of contact: for example, a person administering mouth-to-mouth resuscitation. At present, there is no completely satisfactory prophylactic antibiotic regimen. Regardless of the use of antimicrobial prophylaxis, exposed personnel should report for medical evaluation at the earliest sign of fever or illness.

Postoperative wound infection

Prophylactic antibiotic therapy as ordinarily used cannot be expected to reduce the incidence of postoperative wound infections and is therefore not generally recommended. However, antimicrobial drugs given prophylactically prior to and at the time of injury, and in adequate doses, have been found to decrease the incidence of postoperative wound infection in selected patients. These drugs do not reduce the frequency of respiratory or urinary tract infections among postoperative patients. They should not be used unless there is a significant risk of infection associated with the surgery considered. The results of several well-controlled studies suggest that therapeutic doses of antibiotics, when selected with knowledge of the most common pathogens expected and given only prior to and during the surgical procedure, decrease the incidence of wound infections. This effect has been clearly shown among patients with operations involving the gastrointestinal, genitourinary, or respiratory tracts. Continued administration of antimicrobial therapy after the surgical procedure has been completed is not required, and no increase in complications attributed to antibiotic therapy was noted with this technique.

Staphylococcal postoperative infections have been noted frequently among surgical patients known to be carriers of staphylococci prior to surgery. Treatment to suppress the carrier state has been shown to reduce this risk.

Prophylactic antibiotics, usually methicillin or another penicillinase-resistant antibiotic, such as oxacillin, nafcillin, or cloxacillin, are used routinely by many surgeons for the prevention of endocarditis during and after open-heart operations. The efficacy of this procedure is still under investigation.

Syphilis

If syphilis is diagnosed promptly, and if infected patients are appropriately treated, it rarely should be necessary to administer prophylactic treatment to hospital personnel or to other patients in the hospital. Syphilis can usually be prevented by the administration of procaine or benzathine penicillin G in appropriate doses to persons shortly after exposure. In persons allergic to penicillin, erythromycin or tetracycline can be used. Monthly serologic tests for syphilis are recommended for six months after exposure.

Tuberculosis

If the tuberculin reaction of an employee changes from negative to positive, appropriate evaluation and follow-up is indicated in accordance with the plan in Appendix C, page 171.

STERILIZATION AND DISINFECTION

Developments in medical and surgical practice since the 1950s have greatly complicated considerations of safety to patients, particularly in terms of sterilization and disinfection procedures. Because of interference with patients' immune mechanisms and such procedures as implants in tissues or organs that cannot eliminate invaders of any kind, in many instances no distinction can be made between pathogens and nonpathogens. When such conditions exist, methods of sterilization must be chosen that come as close as possible to the ideal of sterility. When considering such procedures as protective isolation, the choice of methods for disinfection must be made to meet as high a standard as possible.

Sterility, theoretically, is an absolute term indicating that no living organisms or particles exist on or in the article or materials. However, as pointed out by Kelsey, "It is a philosophical concept that can never be unequivocally demonstrated in a real world." The best that can be expected in practice is that the likelihood of an occasional organism surviving the process used is very remote. In effect, the choice of method to be used is not only governed by the idea that the chosen process must be very close to the ideal but is also affected by the magnitude of the risk of using the items if a few contaminants survive. In practice, sterility deals with risk-benefit ratios.

Disinfection refers to the process whereby only certain infectious agents, usually vegetative forms of pathogenic bacteria, are destroyed. Certain stronger agents also destroy spores and therefore are called sporicidal. However, the degree or level of disinfection desired must be considered in terms of safety for the purpose intended.

The term "antiseptic" is useful in medical practice to designate chemicals used to disinfect human or animal tissues.

It follows that those concerned with setting standards and choosing methods need to have a clear concept of at least two levels of sterilization and three levels of disinfection:

Sterilization.
> Level A. The most stringent. In terms of organisms known to be highly resistant to the process, chances of survivors should be lower than one in a million.
>
> Level B. Safe, routine working level. Chances of one survivor should be as close as possible to one in a million but should certainly be better than one in a thousand.

Disinfection.
> Level A. Sporicidal.
> Level B. No vegetative forms resistant.
> Level C. Active against certain types of organisms but not against others.

In all considerations of methods to be used, one basic principle must never be forgotten: *All practical methods for sterilization or disinfection can be overchallenged by grossly dirty and heavily contaminated materials.* Therefore, articles or materials must be thoroughly cleaned before they are processed.

Sterilization

In practice, sterilization is accomplished by exposing articles to dry or moist heat, to the action of chemical agents, or to various types of radiation. Dry heat is not used in hospitals except for the occasional flaming of an instrument, in incinerators, or in laboratories having regulated hot-air ovens. Moist heat is generally preferred. This is used as steam under pressure in autoclaves, with a minimum heating requirement of 121°C. (250°F.) for 15 minutes. The moisture supplied by the steam is essential for sure killing, and therefore each bundle or package must be free from air pockets or seals that can block penetration of moisture. Pressure itself has no influence on bacterial killing; it is used only to attain higher temperatures or to keep fluids from boiling.

Among the chemical agents used for sterilization, it is difficult to find gases or solutions capable of unquestioned sterilization. Evidence is often lacking as to their capability of killing some viruses, such as hepatitis. Nearly all commonly used chemical agents are disinfectants, although very strong alcohol-formaldehyde mixtures, activated glutaraldehyde, very strong acids, and gases such as ethylene oxide or beta propriolactone come close to accomplishing full sterilization. Usually the highest degree of disinfecting ability is judged by action on spores.

Steam sterilization

Steam sterilization is the most certain and the most commonly used method for rendering instruments or materials completely sterile. Its efficiency depends on the penetration of packs by saturated steam at a specified temperature for a specified period of time.

It is generally agreed that exposure to saturated steam at 121° to 123°C. (250° to 254°F.) for 15 to 45 minutes, depending on parcel size and wrapping, accomplishes sterilization without excessive damage to most materials. This method requires the removal of air from within and around the packs and an operating steam pressure of 15 to 17 pounds per square inch.

Many steam pressure sterilizers depend upon gravity displacement of air from the chamber and from within the packs being sterilized for steam penetration to be complete. Improper packing and positioning of the contents of the sterilizer may cause failure of sterilization, even though the pressure gauges and temperature charts indicate that the equipment has been operating correctly. For efficient steam sterilization there must also be proper construction, installation, maintenance, and operation of the autoclave.

In the maintenance of autoclaves, steam outlets and air filtration elements must be cleaned frequently on a regular schedule. Regardless of the efficiency of initial installation and of recording devices, the sterilizing equipment and steam supply should be checked at regular intervals. Autoclaves should be fitted with recording thermometers, even though they record only the steam temperature at the discharge port. There also should be a proper lagging of the steam supply line, and a trap should be inserted close to the apparatus in order to avoid excessively wet steam.

High-vacuum sterilization

Options in technique have been created by the availability of high-vacuum autoclaves. These steam sterilizers create a high degree of vacuum in the chamber once or twice before the steam is admitted and then again after it has been evacuated.

With high-vacuum equipment, the total time of the cycle is considerably reduced. Materials are moistened only for very short periods, and they emerge dry, thereby lessening damage to rubber, fabrics, and sharp instruments. High-vacuum autoclaves have greater tolerances in chamber-packing techniques. There is less danger of creating air pockets, and there is less chance of the steam failing to penetrate to the centers of packs.

The disadvantages are that the equipment is highly complex and calls for expert servicing. Because of the greater steam requirements, it is expensive to buy and to install. There also is a tendency to falsely regard the equipment as entirely foolproof. Experimental work demonstrates a possible concertina-like effect of such high vacuum on air pockets, whereby the air expands and contracts but does not mix with the steam. Other problems are superheating of the surfaces of materials and residual air entrapment within small packages that are part of light loads. Finally, there is still controversy over the degree of vacuum that is necessary. As a guide, the British Ministry of Health has suggested that the equipment is efficient when 98 per cent (0.4 inch, 1.0 centimeter mercury, or 10 torr) or more of the air is removed from the chamber in no longer than five minutes by an oil-sealed pump.

Some high-vacuum equipment uses a water-ring pump that removes 88 to 90 per cent of the air and cycles that vacuum twice before releasing steam. This method is claimed to be as effective as using the very high vacuum, but experimental work does not support this claim.

In general, the relatively high initial cost of the completely automated equipment along with the requirement for highly skilled service have to be balanced against the advantages of timesaving for operators and of reduced damage to fabrics and equipment. At this time, it is not known whether sterilization by the high-vacuum method is superior to sterilization by the gravity displacement system, given proper operation of each.

Sterilization failure

The sterilization procedure may fail as a result of any one of three reasons: First, the equipment or dressings may not have been placed in the sterilizer at all, but may have become mixed with equipment already sterilized. Second, the actual sterilizing may have been inadequate for various reasons, some of which were noted previously. Third, the materials may have become contaminated while in storage.

The first type of failure may be reduced by the use of commercially available indicators, such as adhesive paper on which black stripes appear when it has been exposed to moist heat under pressure. The black stripes indicate that the article wrapped in the adhesive paper has been in the autoclave, although it does not prove that the article is sterile. Color-change glass ampules also indicate that a certain temperature has been attained in the interior of a package. Paper test strips or culture vials contaminated with spores of *Bacillus stearothermophilus,* which is highly resistant to heat, can be included in the pack being sterilized and be bacteriologically tested afterward as a means of determining the sterility of package interiors. These test materials should be placed in the most inaccessible positions, such as the centers of large packs and the fingers of gloves. Tests should be conducted on a variety of articles as frequently as possible, at least once a month. Smaller hospitals can forward the sterilized spore strips and the control strips to a reference laboratory.

The use of a thermocouple or a thermistor is helpful in testing and controlling the steam penetration and interior temperature of articles in a sterilizer. The sensing element is buried in a large test bundle, and the sterilizing cycle is timed so that it will start only when the element records the critical interior temperature, usually 121° to 125°C. (250° to 257°F.).

Packs sterilized in the initial steps of preparation may be contaminated by incoming air during the breaking of the vacuum at the end of the sterilizing cycle. For this reason, the air filter on the inlet should be checked carefully. Some types of filter, such as cellulose fiber, need to be changed as often as once a month, whereas others, such as multiple glass wool discs in cartridges, last at least six months. If sterile but damp packs are placed on nonsterile surfaces, bacteria may penetrate the textile cover and contaminate the contents through the condensate on the wrappings. Thus, if possible, packs should be allowed to cool on the sterilizer carriage.

Despite modern refinement in automatic control equipment, the human element is still the determining factor in the reliability of autoclaving. Supervisors and operators must be familiar with the basic principles of the process and must have detailed instruction in all phases of operation, as well as a manual for reference.

Ethylene oxide sterilization

Studies by Phillips, Kaye, and others established the fact that ethylene oxide is a useful chemical agent for destroying pathogenic bacteria on surfaces of certain porous materials. Moreover, it does so at comparatively low temperatures and without corroding or otherwise damaging a wide variety of materials sensitive to high heat or to other chemical bactericides. Ethylene oxide was used extensively to preserve foodstuffs and as an insecticide prior to World War II, but not until then were its medical possibilities explored. Industrial usage grew rapidly following the description of its use for sterilizing plastic bandages.

The slow killing action of ethylene oxide cannot be accelerated beyond that achieved at a concentration of 900 milligrams per liter at temperatures over 37°C. (98.6°F.). Evidence suggests that the gas must be in solution at the cell surface in order for it to pass into the bacterial cell and achieve its killing effect. Spores are slightly more resistant than vegetative forms of bacteria. Bacteria such as *Mycobacterium tuberculosis* are relatively resistant, probably because of their waxy coatings. Ethylene oxide is highly soluble in water and can permeate oils, organic solvents, rubber, neoprene, and many plastics with relative ease, although the role of intrinsic moisture in these materials is not fully understood.

Various characteristics of ethylene oxide have been defined with respect to its value as a sterilizing agent of medical supplies. Some of its more important characteristics are as follows. If bacteria or spores have survived a stringent desiccation, they may not be killed by the gas, usually because they are protected inside crystals or protein conglomerates. Also, rehydration of such microorganisms by the relative humidity of the surrounding atmosphere is a difficult and slow process. Further, certain metals, particularly magnesium, zinc, and tin, combine with moist ethylene oxide to form a glutinous gel; a few chemicals, such as chromic acid or its derivatives, bind or inactivate the gas. Wrapping materials that are highly permeable to ethylene oxide include paper, cloth, nonlaminated (monoextruded) and polyethylene film; wrapping materials to be avoided because of impermeability include linear-type nylon, Mylar®, aluminum laminates, and laminated (coextruded) polyethylene films. Although ethylene oxide appears to diffuse through and around equipment or materials with comparative ease, its basic action is probably that of heavy gas displacing air, combined with extreme solubility in any retained moisture. Gas concentrations at the top of a chamber may be below minimum requirements.

To minimize explosion hazards, ethylene oxide is supplied as 10 to 12 per cent of the gas in an inert vehicle, such as Freon or carbon dioxide. In order to reach effective concentrations in the chamber (at least 450 milligrams per liter), it is necessary to remove most of the air first by creating a vacuum.

The systemic toxicity of ethylene oxide is low, and its effects are easily reversible. The maximum allowable concentration in a working space should not exceed 50 parts per million. Ethylene oxide in high concentrations irritates mucous membranes and skin, depresses the central nervous system, and can cause liver and kidney damage. When the gas is in solution or is bound to such materials as rubber or chromic-tanned leather, it may cause skin vesication or inflammation of mucous membranes. Therefore, such materials must be well aerated before being allowed to come into contact with the skin; several days of aeration may be required for certain heavy porous materials. For further details, the report by Matsumoto is recommended.

The use of ethylene oxide in hospital practice requires certain safeguards and attention to details. For example, it is not safe to desiccate articles for sterilization in a forced-draft hot-air apparatus or to dry them over a heating coil when the ambient relative humidity of the room air is low. In one series of failures of rubber glove sterilization, it was found that the glove-drying and powdering machine was too efficient: The nondesiccated, spore-impregnated test strips inserted into the gloves before ethylene oxide treatment were sterilized, whereas dried materials washed out of the gloves contained large numbers of viable bacteria.

Some types of equipment, particularly small units, may not be designed to provide adequate control of humidity. In well-designed sterilizers, the prevacuum, the raised temperature of the chamber, the arrangements for mobilizing the nonflammable ethylene oxide gas mixture, and the humidification function as guards against the dangers of the failures described previously. If a new, highly specialized piece of equipment is acquired, the manufacturers should be consulted about the possibility of its being damaged by ethylene oxide. Similar consultation should be made with respect to wrapping materials, particularly new types of plastics.

Although test strips definitely should be used, it is not wise to depend completely on test strips of cultured bacteria in sample packages for judging the efficacy of the ethylene oxide sterilization. Such procedures are reliable for steam sterilization, but for ethylene oxide there are too many variables. For example, test strips are not rendered too dry for ethylene oxide action, but some of the equipment in the chamber may be. It is necessary, therefore, that checks for efficiency include samplings from equipment known to have some degree of contamination before exposure. Such sampling is particularly important if changes are made in the methods of washing, drying, or preparing articles prior to sterilization.

Changes in packaging should be tested also. Control samples should be identical in kind and in manner of preparation to those being sterilized. For example, a length of tubing of the same material and bore as a bronchoscope or other scope, washed, dried, and wrapped by the same process as the other scopes, can be processed as a control sample for scopes being sterilized.

In summary, failures or undesirable side effects of sterilization with ethylene oxide must be guarded against by ensuring that:

- Materials in the equipment are not harmed by the gas.
- Wrappings or other coverings are permeable to the gas.
- Materials or equipment are not rendered excessively dry prior to sterilization.
- The effectiveness of the process is checked routinely at least once a week by:
  1. Placing spore-strips in larger packages at the bottom *and at the top* of a load, culturing afterward to make certain that the packages have been sterilized.
  2. Sampling each type of equipment (or mock-ups of each type) for sterility.
  3. Daily using capsules that change color when exposed to the gas. These capsules are similar to tapes that blacken when exposed to steam.
- Materials that retain the gas or gas products are aerated for adequate periods before being released for use.

Radiation sterilization

Radiation sterilization currently is not a routine hospital procedure. However, a rapidly advancing technology may, in the near future, result in the designing and marketing of smaller, economically feasible units. Members of infection control committees may find it useful to have a reasonable understanding of the radiation sterilization processes used by commercial purveyors of sterile articles. Commercial plants for sterilization by radiation are becoming available. For a full discussion, readers are referred to the bibliography.

Radiation can be divided into nonionizing and ionizing. Of the nonionizing types, ultrasonic waves disrupt cells, infrared rays kill by producing heat, and ultraviolet rays interfere with cell metabolism. These agents can be used to produce sterility for certain purposes, but their applicability is strictly limited. The most commonly used type of nonionizing radiation is ultraviolet irradiation. It is used for reducing viral or bacterial counts in air, but it is very difficult to use for true sterilization.

Of the ionizing types of radiation, high-energy electrons from accelerators or electromagnetic gamma rays are used. Each has advantages and disadvantages.

High-energy electron plants require little space; safety precautions are not elaborate; and sterilization is achieved quickly, in seconds. On the other hand, penetration is poor and only small packages can be processed. Above certain dosage levels, radioactivity may be induced in articles being processed. Further, maintenance of constant, standard dosage is difficult.

Of the heavy, particulate radiations, gamma rays are the most suitable for sterilization for various reasons, including their inability to induce radioactivity in materials exposed to them. The most commonly used source is cobalt-60, but for smaller units cesium-137 with its longer half-life and lesser need for shielding may have advantages. Gamma irradiation is advantageous because the emission is dependably constant and the type of ray is well defined. There is good penetrating power, and suitably designed plants can process relatively large packages; such plants are able to operate continuously with a minimum of attention from staff. Gamma irradiation is disadvantageous because exposure times are long, from 36 to 48 hours, and plants are relatively elaborate and expensive.

Because of constancy of emission, cobalt-60 plants facilitate accurate dosage schedules and dependable predictions of the killing effects for different types of microorganisms and viruses. Dosage schedules are quoted in megarads (Mrads) for sterilization, and in kilorads for what might be termed "disinfection" or "decontamination" of ordinarily sensitive bacteria. Some relatively rare, highly resistant bacteria, such as *Streptococcus faecium,* may need 3- to 4-Mrad dosage for 10^{-6} (99.999 per cent) certainty of kill. The lethal effects for larger viruses, such as vaccinia, tend to fall below the 2-Mrad range, and for the smallest viruses, such as some encephalitis viruses or foot-and-mouth disease virus, requirements may go as high as 5 Mrads. Although controversy still exists in European countries, a 2.5-Mrad dosage for such articles as disposable syringes and needles appears to be adequate provided there are few contaminants prior to sterilization.

Ionizing radiation, in general, shows an exponential relationship between dose and effect. Hence, reliable predictions of kill can be made. There is no appreciable temperature elevation during treatment, but some textiles are weakened and some plastics are adversely affected. In terms of medical supplies, the main advantage is that articles can be packaged in impermeable containers or wrappings before sterilization, because no vapor or gas has to penetrate the packages. This gives the articles an indefinite shelf life.

It has been pointed out that certainty of kill can be determined with reasonable accuracy for radiation processes, but as for *all other sterilization methods in common use, an excessive challenge can always overcome the system*. Basically, articles or materials prepared and packaged prior to exposure to the process must be carefully controlled in terms of general cleanliness and freedom from gross contamination by microorganisms.

Disinfection

Although the term disinfection implies incomplete destruction of living organisms, some disinfecting processes can be used in such concentrated form or for such long periods that sterilization can be achieved. Other disinfecting processes can never achieve sterilization.

The processes in common use can be classed as physical agents or as chemical agents. Heat and radiation are examples of physical agents. As for chemical agents, there is such a vast number available that only group characteristics can be reviewed within the scope of this handbook.

Physical agents

Although two kinds of heat, dry and moist, can be classed as physical agents, dry heat is not routinely used for disinfection. However, moist heat, directed at the destruction of vegetative forms of bacteria, parasites, and mycotic agents, is commonly used in various ways: rinsing dishes with water at 82°C. (180°F.) or more for five minutes; washing laundry in water at 71°C. (160°F.) for 10 to 25 minutes; ironing or pressing with steam at 160°C. (320°F.); and placing articles in boiling water or directing steam at them for five minutes. For all temperatures below the boiling point, a minimum time for killing pathogens must be considered. The lowest useful temperatures are in the range of pasteurization, 65.5°C. (150°F.) for 30 minutes.

The other type of physical agent used for disinfection, ultraviolet (UV) radiation, can kill nearly all disease-producing organisms, provided the rays impinge upon the organisms with sufficient intensity for the minimum time required. In actual practice, difficulties with this process stem from four basic characteristics:
- UV rays have very limited penetration, and organisms are easily protected within dust particles, dried mucus, and so forth.
- UV rays lose strength rapidly as they pass through air or water surrounding the source tube. In water, the intensity is reduced to 38 per cent at a distance of 2 inches from the tube. In air, the intensity is reduced to 25 per cent at a distance of 8 to 9 inches.
- UV ray emissions from tubes are markedly reduced by fine films of dust, moisture, or oily substances on the glass surface.
- The emission of UV rays from the tube source in the lethal range (2,500 to 2,600 A.) gradually weakens, without any discernible change in visible-light emissions.

Because of these difficulties associated with ultraviolet irradiation, the conditions of use have to be carefully controlled, and the equipment regularly serviced and monitored with UV meters. Another limiting factor in the general use of UV irradiation is the ease with which it causes conjunctivitis or burns of human skin.

Much thought and engineering skill have been devoted to designing portable units or installations that reduce counts of airborne or waterborne bacteria, mainly by guiding air or water streams close to high-intensity UV sources. Studies have been made of the effect of fixed sources with natural air circulation passing room air close enough to the tubes for bacterial killing.

Extensive studies have not encouraged general usage of UV radiation in hospitals. However, there is some evidence of slight reductions in wound infections in "refined clean" cases of neurosurgery, and there are strong advocates for its use in tuberculosis treatment areas.

Chemical agents

Many groups of chemical compounds or elements destroy some living cells, protoplasts, and viruses. When chemicals are used for killing infective agents, the following principles should be kept in mind.

In order to kill, the chemical must penetrate the cell wall and the cellular substance; it can do so only in the form of a solution that surrounds and penetrates the cell. Therefore, any infectious agent that survives complete desiccation of its surroundings as a spore or that is protected from moisture by being within an impervious substance, such as a crystal or inspissated protein, will resist being killed by a chemical agent.

Every chemical agent used for disinfection requires time to kill, and each exerts its maximal effect at a concentration that is not necessarily the strongest obtainable. For example, ethanol in a 70 per cent concentration is more effective than at a 90 or 95 per cent concentration. Moreover, the nearer the concentration to the optimum, the shorter the time required for the killing effect. Temperature also affects killing action, and in many instances chemical lethality increases markedly with small increments in temperature.

Chemical disinfectants affect pathogenic agents unequally. Some may be so ineffective under certain circumstances that microorganisms can thrive in them, as evidenced by the growth of the tubercle bacillus or pseudomonas in some aqueous solutions of quaternary ammonium compounds. It should be recognized, therefore, that no disinfectant is universally effective.

When formaldehyde vapor is used with steam in a chamber kept at 80°C. (176°F.), almost complete sterility is achieved. The difficulty of ensuring formaldehyde diffusion into and around all articles, particularly small-bore tubing, can be solved by drawing repeated (usually three) vacuum levels. Similarly, acid glutaraldehyde in water is just as active as the alkalinized (activated) glutaraldehyde at temperatures over 40°C. (104°F.).

All chemical disinfectants can be neutralized or weakened by contact with various substances. Some are readily neutralized by proteinaceous materials; others are inactivated by some soaps and detergents or by metals of containers, such as aluminum. These incompatibilities must be known to the users, and disinfecting mixtures must be prepared only by pharmacists or chemists who have knowledge of these facts.

Many disinfectants, particularly quaternary ammonium compounds, only restrict bacterial growth in high dilutions but can kill bacteria when used in much stronger solutions. Some disinfectants adhere to bacteria and will not wash off, and thereby prevent growth in laboratory tests even though the bacteria have not been killed. Laboratory techniques, therefore, must include neutralization of such chemicals, particularly in the testing of iodine.

For details of optimal concentrations and for lists of the many chemical compounds available as disinfectants, reference must be made to textbooks. Within the scope of this handbook, only a list of the principal groups and their properties can be offered (see Table 8, page 106).

Because chemical disinfectants are active compounds and can have adverse effects on component parts or materials in instruments or equipment, chemical incompatibilities must be known. Therefore, the following features must govern the use of a particular chemical disinfectant:
- The nature and composition of the object to be disinfected must be known in order to avoid damage.
- The certainty with which the object can be freed from all kinds of dirt must also be known. It is necessary to know whether there may be a residue, the nature of such residue, and which chemical agents it might neutralize.
- It is also necessary to know the most important pathogenic agents to be destroyed and the limits of the disinfection desired.

For example, spore formers are usually not important on dishes or proctoscopes. Tubercle bacilli are of major importance only in specific instances. The optimal care of the environment of a patient isolated for typhoid fever requires a different disinfectant (a phenolic) from that of a patient isolated for a staphylococcal infection (a quaternary). The strength, temperature, and time of contact that are practical for the particular technique of cleaning must also be known, in addition to such factors as strength of the disinfectant appropriate for operators who wear gloves. The human tendency to rinse off odoriferous or irritating disinfectants too soon after application must also be considered.

In the overall use of disinfectants, unavoidable incompatibilities may be found, including such actions as removal of hexachlorophene by alcohol, weakening of quaternary ammonium compounds by cottons and soaps, and neutralizing of iodine by aluminum surfaces. The possibilities that overdesiccation might prevent effective use of formaldehyde gas or ethylene oxide, or that ineffective rinsing or covering might cause release or leakage of irritating or toxic agents, must be kept in mind. No laboratory test can foretell the efficiency of a disinfectant for use in the hospital, because the conditions of use cannot be properly duplicated in the laboratory. Standardized laboratory tests are helpful guides, but the real test of effectiveness comes only by actual use. Also, the question of comparative costs must be considered in the choice of effective disinfectants. Recommended procedures of known effectiveness are shown in Table 9, page 108.

Antisepsis

Antiseptics are intended for use on or in human tissues and only rarely can be used in concentrations strong enough to kill bacteria quickly. Some have direct, relatively fast killing effects, but in most cases the essential

Table 8
EVALUATION OF USEFUL ANTIMICROBIAL CHEMICALS

Compound (chemical group and subgroup)	Usual activity against bacteria					Speed of bacterial killing		Inactivation by proteins or mucus	Other Characteristics
	Gram-pos.	Most gram-neg.	Proteus and Pseudo.	TB	Spores	Maximum strength	Antiseptic strength		
1. ALCOHOLS	Good	Good	Good	Fair	None	+++	+++	***	Use on tissues limited to skin; optimal strengths 60-80%
2. PHENOLS, CRESOLS	Fair	Good	Good	Fair	Poor	+++	+++	****	Only for necrotic tissues
a. Synthetics and chlorophenols	Good	Good	Fair	Fair	Poor	+++	+ to +++	***	Weak solutions do not irritate but some sensitize
3. ALDEHYDES									
a. Formaldehyde	Good	Good	Good	Good	Fair	++++	Corrosive	****	Corrosive, irritating to tissues
b. Glutaraldehyde	Good	Good	Good	Good	Good	+++	++	**	Some irritation, possible sensitization
4. SURFACE-ACTIVE AGENTS									
a. Quaternary ammoniums	Good	Fair	Very poor	None	None	+ to +++	+ to ++	*	Some types with little action on gram-negatives
b. Amphoteric series compounds (Tegos)	Fair	Good	Good	Fair	Poor	+	0	**	Inactivated by many chemicals
5. IODINE, PURE	Good	Good	Good	Good	Fair	++++	++++	***	Tissue usage limited to skin and some mucous membranes
a. Iodophors	Good	Good	Good	Fair	None	+++	+++	**	No skin "burns"; no staining of fabrics

6. CHLORINE, FREE	Fair	Good	Good	Fair	Fair	+++	Corrosive	****	Not usable on or in tissues
a. Chloramines	Fair	Good	Good	Poor	Poor	+++	+	**	Some effect on tissues
7. METALS, IONIC (Hg, Ag, Sn, Cu)	Fair	Good	Good	None	None	++	++	****	Use on tissues very limited (protein coagulants)
a. Thimerosal (Merthiolate)	Good	Good	Good	None	Very poor	++	++	***	Strongly static, like a dye
8. ACRIDINES, FLAVINES	Good	Good	Good	Fair	None	Poor	+	0	0	Tissue toxicity very low; occasional sensitization
a. With sulfas	Good	Good	Good	None	Poor	+	+	0	Same
9. CHLOROGUANIDINES (chlorhexidine)	Good	Good	Good	Fair	None	++	++	*	No tissue toxicity or sensitizing effects
10. SOME COMBINATIONS									
a. 1 and 5	Very good	Very good	Good	Fair	Fair	++++	++++	***	Fastest killing of bacteria on skin surfaces
b. 1 and 3	Good	Good	Good	Good	Good	++++	Corrosive	***	Corrosive and irritating
c. 1, 2, and 3	Very good	Very good	Very good	Good	Good	++++	Corrosive	**	Corrosive and irritating
d. 4 and 9	Good	Good	Fair	Poor	None	++	++	*	Some chemicals like soaps weaken action
e. 4 and 8	Good	Good	Poor	None	None	+	+	*	For skin and wounds but no action on pseudomonas

Killing: 0, static; +, slow; ++, moderate; +++, rapid; ++++, almost immediate.
Inactivation: 0, none; *, minimal; **, appreciable; ***, quite marked; ****, very extensive.

action is bacteriostatic, the stopping of microbial growth. Eventual elimination of infecting agents in bacteriostasis depends upon prevention of bacterial reproduction, dying of older bacteria, mechanical removal of

Table 9
RECOMMENDATIONS FOR CHEMICAL DISINFECTION AND STERILIZATION OF INSTRUMENTS

Equipment	Disinfecting treatment		Sterilizing treatment
	Category A	Category B	Category C
Smooth, hard objects	1A for 10 min. 2 for 5 min. 3 for 10 min. 4A for 10 min. 5A for 5 min.‖ 6A for 5 min. 8 for 5 min. 9 for 5 min.	1B for 15 min. 2 for 10 min. 4B for 20 min. 5B for 20 min. 6B for 20 min.§ 8 for 15 min. 9 for 15 min.	2 for 18 hr. 7 for 3-12 hr.‡ 8 for 12 hr. 9 for 10 hr.
Rubber tubing and catheters, completely filled	3 for 10 min. 4A for 10 min. 5A for 5 min.	4B for 20 min. 5B for 20 min. 9 for 15 min.	7 for 3-12 hr.‡
Polyethylene tubing and catheters, completely filled	1A for 10 min. 3 for 10 min. 4A for 10 min. 5A for 10 min.	1B for 15 min. 4B for 20 min. 5B for 20 min. 9 for 15 min.	2 for 12 hr. 7 for 3-12 hr.‡ 8 for 12 hr. 9 for 10 hr.
Lensed instruments	3 for 10 min. 4A for 10 min. 5A for 10 min.	8 for 15 min. 9 for 15 min.	7 for 3-12 hr.‡ 8 for 12 hr. 9 for 10 hr.
Thermometers, oral and rectal‖	1C for 10 min.	1C for 15 min.	2 for 12 hr. 7 for 3-12 hr.‡ 8 for 12 hr. 9 for 10 hr.
Hinged instruments#	1A for 15 min. 2 for 10 min. 3 for 20 min. 4A for 20 min. 5A for 15 min. 8 for 10 min. 9 for 10 min.	1B for 20 min. 2 for 15 min. 4B for 30 min. 5B for 30 min. 8 for 20 min. 9 for 20 min.	7 for 3-12 hr.‡ 8 for 12 hr. 9 for 10 hr.
Inhalation and anesthesia equipment	1A for 15 min. 3 for 20 min. 9 for 5 min.	1B for 20 min. 9 for 20 min.	7 for 3-12 hr.‡ 9 for 10 hr.

This table was contributed by Earle H. Spaulding, Temple University, Philadelphia, and George F. Mallison, Center for Disease Control, Atlanta, as submitted to the American Society for Microbiology's ad hoc Committee on Microbiological Standards of Disinfection in Hospitals.
*Time required depends on procedure used.
†Not recommended for metal instruments.
‡Preferably washed with soap and water and thoroughly wiped before disinfection or sterilization. Alcohol-iodine solutions remove markings on poor-grade thermometers.
§Must first be cleansed in order to be free of organic salt.

Key to chemical compounds:

1A   70-90% Ethyl alcohol or isopropyl alcohol*
1B   70-90% Ethyl alcohol
1C   Compound 1 plus 0.2% iodine
2   20% Formalin plus 70% alcohol solution*
3   1:500 Aqueous quaternary ammonium solution*
4A   Iodophor (100 ppm available iodine)*
4B   Iodophor (500 ppm available iodine)*
5A   1% Aqueous phenolic solution*
5B   2% Aqueous phenolic solution*
6A   Sodium hypochlorite (100 ppm available chlorine)
6B   Sodium hypochlorite (1,000 ppm available chlorine)
7   Ethylene oxide gas
8   20% Aqueous formalin
9   2% Aqueous activated glutaraldehyde*

Key to categories of microorganisms:

A   Vegetative bacteria and fungi, influenza viruses
B   A plus tubercle bacilli, enteroviruses
C   A plus B plus hepatitis viruses,† bacterial and some fungal spores

---

‖To prevent corrosion, 0.2% sodium nitrite should be present in alcohols, formalin, formaldehyde-alcohol, quaternary ammonium, and iodophor solutions, and 0.5% sodium bicarbonate should be present in phenolic situations.
#Very little direct observation has been possible; use heat whenever possible.

bacteria from the site, and such biological reactions as phagocytosis and bacteriolysis by body fluids. Antiseptics that can be used with complete safety in or on delicate tissue are nearly always purely bacteriostatic. However, some used for eliminating bacteria from skin surfaces in hand scrubs, preoperative preps, and so forth can be tolerated in bactericidal concentrations. Certain types of chemicals also can be used at bactericidal levels in the urinary bladder or the large bowel, but other usage is essentially bacteriostatic. For skin surfaces, iodine in alcohol is still the best all-around antiseptic.

Criteria for selecting the type of antiseptic and its strength should be based on the antimicrobial spectrum of the agent, the types of bacteria to be eliminated, the speed of bactericidal action in relation to the time bacteria are liable to be exposed to the agent, and the tissue to which it will be applied. Also, factors or materials that are liable to weaken or neutralize the chemical agent, for example, various proteins, mucus, ionized elements, acid or alkaline pH ranges, must be considered.

Since 1972, toxicity data involving new concepts of absorption of antiseptics or disinfectants through unbroken skin have elicited questions of safe usage. In the case of hexachlorophene, further studies are being carried out, but it is generally agreed that this antiseptic should be used on newborn infants only after careful consideration of the need. Reinvestigations of other antiseptics are proceeding.

The notes in Table 8, page 106, focus more on tissue damage than on pharmacological toxicity. Highly irritating antiseptics, such as Dakin's solution, may be very useful for cleaning up dirty, necrotic areas. Groups such as the phenols, synthetic phenols, chlorophenols, and the quaternary ammonium compounds represent such a vast multiplicity of chemical types, each with slightly different spectra of antibacterial action, that Table 8 can state only an approximation of the group characteristics.

Scouring powders or bleaches that contain chlorine are useful in decontaminating bathtubs, washbasins, and so forth. The chlorine content of the brand used should be verified. Immersion of equipment in a solution of 1,000 parts per million chlorine is often a satisfactory method of decontaminating items that are impractical to sterilize by steam. A suitable solution can be prepared by adding about 3 ounces of liquid household bleach to one gallon of water. For heavily contaminated articles or to guard against transfer of hepatitis virus, 10 times this strength is advised.

A disinfectant for housekeeping purposes or for decontaminating instruments may be the source of a great deal of trouble if it is a skin irritant, tends to sensitize users, or causes dermatitis or other reactions. Thus, in specific instances decisions must be made between a stronger bactericidal disinfectant that is so irritating to the skin that it must be removed soon after application and a weaker, nonirritating disinfectant that need not be removed and has ample time to act.

In considering disinfectants for instruments to be used in the respiratory or gastrointestinal tract, a choice must be made between a stronger, quicker acting disinfectant that would damage the mucosa unless the instruments are thoroughly rinsed and a weaker, less effective disinfectant that does not irritate or damage the mucosa and thus requires no rinsing. Factors such as rinsing or extra handling, which increase chances of recontamination after disinfection, must be considered also.

HAND WASHING

Hand washing is absolutely essential for prevention and control of nosocomial infection; there is no substitute for it. Moreover, hand washing is a procedure that must be practiced faithfully by all hospital personnel without exception. It should be purposefully and efficiently performed by all personnel in accordance with instructions recommended by the infection control committee.

Hand washing in its simplest form is merely a procedure for cleansing the hands and wrists—and under some specifications, the forearms, and elbows—in order to remove foreign matter, including transient microorganisms. Depending on the technique used, some of the surface materials—notably the sebum, sweat, skin cells, and body hairs—are also removed and some residue of the cleaning agent remains on the surface of the skin. In the hospital, however, hand washing means much more. It represents the most effective method for preventing transfer of infection to the patient, from one patient to another, from a patient to hospital personnel, and from one part of the patient's body to another.

Aids

Soaps and other detergents aid in the cleansing processes through their properties of wetting, penetration, emulsification, deflocculation, preferential wetting, and dispersion.

The addition of antimicrobial chemicals to soaps and detergents can selectively improve the killing of certain pathogenic bacteria. Thus, for many years the fear of spreading pathogenic staphylococci prompted the routine use of hexachlorophene in detergents and soaps. Other agents, for example, 70 per cent alcohol rinses and iodophors, have been used for less specific purposes. Evidence of hexachlorophene toxicity in newborn infants has prompted reexamination of toxic, allergenic, or other undesirable effects when hexachlorophene or other agents are used frequently. For example, the evidence indicating rare photosensitization by the halogenated salicylanilides is considered by some authorities to be a contraindication for routine usage.

There appear to be advantages to using antimicrobials in hand washing when heavy contamination is present. However, no advantages exist under ordinary, nonepidemic conditions. It is preferred that soap or detergent be used without antimicrobial additives when no specific problems exist. If special action is needed, alcohol rinsing, iodophors, or hexachlorophene should be considered.

To facilitate cleanliness, the fingernails should be kept closely trimmed. A manicure stick should be used to remove visible dirt, as is done routinely in a complete surgical scrub. Hand brushes and fingernail brushes facilitate the cleansing process by mechanical action, as in preparation scrubbing. Brushes must be soft enough to avoid abrasion of the skin. They must be sterilized at intervals and kept free from bacterial contamination.

Techniques

The extent of hand washing varies with conditions. For example, a prolonged wash, using a soft brush, may be necessary upon starting work or for marked soiling. The use of an orangewood stick or the blunt end of a toothpick may be required, together with solvents or other special measures, for removal of the stains or chemical products used in a hospital.

Hand washing presents certain inconveniences because of the time it requires and its effects on the skin. The techniques used should satisfy the criteria of effectiveness, economy of time and effort, economy of supplies and equipment, comfort, cosmetic appeal, and simplicity. Jewelry should not be worn while hands are washed.

The 10-minute surgical scrub includes washing above the elbows, a germicidal rinse (as with 70 per cent alcohol), and the use of sterile towels. This type of scrub is indicated also for personnel coming on duty in the newborn nursery.

A standard two-minute wash should be demonstrated. The demonstration should show the sequences of wetting, soaping, rinsing; applying friction to all surfaces of hands and forearms, including between the fingers, with and without the use of fingernail stick and brush; drying adequately; and optional use of noncontaminated lotions. The lotion source should be checked periodically, and disposable containers should be used. Emphasis should be placed on technique rather than on rigid procedural or timing requirements. Another useful demonstration is bacteriological sampling and testing before and after handwashing procedures, to show effects of techniques and chemical agents. Sampling is also helpful for the instruction of personnel and as an indicator of compliance with instructions.

At the discretion of the infection control committee, cleansing pads and chemical solutions for use without water may be recommended for hand cleansing in some situations. Individually packaged pads are available, and gauze pads soaked in 70 per cent alcohol are effective as occasional substitutes for scrubbing. Personnel should be informed, however, that even a

10- to 15-second wash will reduce transient skin bacteria significantly.

Facilities for hand washing should be located as conveniently as possible, because proximity is conducive to their greater use. Paper towels should be available, even though single-use or disposable towels may also be provided. The soap dispensers, brushes, sticks for nail cleaning, towel racks, and germ-free lotions should all be conveniently placed.

In some circumstances, such as emergencies, clean or sterile gloves may be used without previous hand washing. It should be remembered, however, that long-time experience in surgery has demonstrated that both hand washing and sterile gloves are essential to achieve asepsis.

Hospital personnel should wash hands:
- When coming on duty.
- When the hands are obviously soiled.
- Between handling of individual patients.
- Before contact about the face and mouth of patients.
- After personal use of the toilet.
- After blowing or wiping the nose.
- On leaving an isolation area or after handling articles from an isolation area.
- After handling used dressings, used sputum containers, soiled urinals, catheters, and bedpans.
- Before eating.
- On completion of duty.

BIBLIOGRAPHY

ARCHITECTURAL CONSIDERATIONS

Carpets

Anderson, R. L. Biological evaluation of carpeting. *Appl. Microbiol.* 18:180, Aug. 1969.

Carpeting versus resilient floor coverings. *Consumer Bull.* 49:29, Mar. 1966.

Cihlar, C. Ohio nursing home fire: an analysis. *Hospitals, J.A.H.A.* 44:2a, Mar. 1, 1970.

Greco, J. T. Carpeting vs. resilient flooring. *Hospitals, J.A.H.A.* 39:55, June 16, 1965.

Parks, G. M. *The Economics of Carpeting and Resilient Flooring. An Evaluation and Comparison.* Philadelphia: Wharton School of Finance and Commerce, Industrial Research Unit, University of Pennsylvania, 1966.

Shaffer, J. G., and Key, I. D. A three year study of carpeting in a general hospital. *Health Lab. Sci.* 6:215, Oct. 1969.

Shaffer, J. G., and others. High-power vacuum keeps bacteria low in care of carpeting. *Mod. Hosp.* 107:166, Oct. 1966.

Unidirectional (laminar) clean airflow

Agnew, B. *The Laminar Flow Clean Room Handbook.* 3rd ed. Garden Grove, Calif.: Agnew-Higgins, Inc., 1968.

Burke, J. F. A bacteria controlled nursing unit and individual patient isolation facility. In: *Proceedings of the International Conference on Nosocomial Infections.* Chicago: American Hospital Association, 1971, pp. 216-19.

Contamination Control Handbook (Pub. SP-5076). Washington, D.C.: National Aeronautics and Space Administration, Technology Utilization Division, Office of Technology Utilization, 1969.

Contamination Control Principles. Washington, D.C.: National Aeronautics and Space Administration, Technology Utilization Division, Office of Technology Utilization, 1967.

Coriell, L. L., and McGarrity, G. J. Elimination of airborne bacteria in the laboratory and operating room. *Bull. Parenteral Drug Assn.* 21:46, Mar.-Apr. 1967.

Fox, D. G. *A Study of the Application of Laminar Flow Ventilation to Operating Rooms* (Public Health Monograph No. 78, PHS No. 1894). Washington, D.C.: U.S. Government Printing Office, 1969.

Goodrich, E. O., and others. Laminar clean air flow in operating rooms. *Bull. Amer. Coll. Surg.* 58:9, July 1973.

Laufman, H. Current status of special air-handling systems in operating rooms. *Med. Instrumentation.* 7:7, Jan.-Feb. 1973.

Noble, W. C., and others. The size distribution of airborne particles carrying microorganisms. *J. Hyg.* (Cambridge) 61:385, Dec. 1963.

Porter, K. W. Laminar flow comes under attack. *Hospitals, J.A.H.A.* 46:142, Oct. 16, 1972.

Riley, R. L., and others. Infectiousness of air from a tuberculosis ward. Ultraviolet irradiation of infected air: comparative infectiousness of different patients. *Amer. Rev. Resp. Dis.* 85:511, Apr. 1962.

Special air systems for operating rooms. *Bull. Amer. Coll. Surg.* 57:18, May 1972.

Wells, W. F. On air-borne infection. Study II. Droplets and droplet nuclei. *Amer. J. Hyg.* 20:611, Nov. 1934.

Whitcomb, J. G., and Clapper, W. E. Ultraclean operating room. *Amer. J. Surg.* 112:681, Nov. 1966.

Whitfield, W. J. State of the art (contamination control) and laminar air-flow concept: Conference on clean room specifications. Reprint No. SCR-652. Albuquerque, N.Mex.: Sandia Corp., May 1963.

ENVIRONMENTAL CONTROL

Duguid, J. P., and Wallace, A. T. Air infection with dust liberated from clothing. *Lancet.* 2:845, Nov. 27, 1948.

Fincher, E. L. Air sampling: application, methods, recommendations. In: *Control of Infection in Hospitals.* Ann Arbor, Mich.: University of Michigan School of Public Health, 1966.

──────────. Surface sampling: application, methods, recommendations. In: *Control of Infection in Hospitals.* Ann Arbor, Mich.: University of Michigan School of Public Health, 1966.

Gonzaga, A. J. Transmission of staphylococci by fomites. *J. Amer. Med. Assn.* 189:711, Sept. 7, 1964.

Hall, L. B. Air sampling for hospitals. *Hosp. Top.* 40:97, June 1962.

Hall, L. B., and Hartnett, J. J. Measurement of the bacterial contamination on surfaces in hospitals. *Pub. Health Rep.* 79:1021, Nov. 1964.

Mallison, G. F. Introduction to microbiology of the institutional environment. In: *Proceedings of the Fourth Annual Technical Meeting of the American Association for Contamination Control.* 6-1:1, May 1965. Boston: AACC, 1965.

Rammelkamp Jr., C. H. Prophylaxis of bacterial disease with antimicrobial drugs. *Amer. J. Med.* 39:804, Nov. 1965.

Riley, R. L. Editorial: The hazard is relative. *Amer. Rev. Resp. Dis.* 96:623, Oct. 1967.

──────────────. J. Burns Amberson Lecture: Aerial dissemination of pulmonary tuberculosis. *Amer. Rev. Tuberculosis.* 76:931, Dec. 1957.

Riley, R. L., and others. Aerial dissemination of pulmonary tuberculosis: a two-year study of contagion in a tuberculosis ward. *Amer. J. Hyg.* 70:185, Sept. 1959.

──────────────. Air hygiene in tuberculosis: quantitative studies of infectivity and control in a pilot ward. *Amer. Rev. Tuberculosis.* 75:420, Mar. 1957.

ISOLATION TECHNIQUES AND PROCEDURES

National Tuberculosis and Respiratory Disease Association. *Infectiousness of Tuberculosis.* New York: NTA, 1967.

Beal, C. B. Plastic bubble isolates patient anywhere in hospital. *Mod. Hosp.* 104:83, Jan. 1965.

Briggs, F. R. Implementing modern concepts of isolation care. *Hospitals, J.A.H.A.* 40:87, May 1, 1966.

Haynes, B. W., and Hency, M. E. Hospital isolation system for preventing cross contamination by staphylococcal and pseudomonas organisms in burn wounds. *Ann. Surg.* 162:641, Oct. 1965.

Kunin, C. M., and Henley, R. W. Isolation procedures for the community hospital: Virginia. *J. Amer. Med. Assn.* 200:295, Apr. 24, 1967.

Landy, J. J. Treatment of the burned patient: use of the germ-free plastic isolator as a barrier against hospital pathogens. *Southern Med. J.* 98:1884, Oct. 1963.

Levenson, S. M., and others. Application of the technology of the germfree laboratory to special problems of patient care. *Amer. J. Surg.* 107:710, May 1964.

Reimer, A. O., and Tillotson, J. L. Food service procedures for reverse isolation. *J. Amer. Diet. Assn.* 48:381, May 1966.

Seidler, F. M. Adapting nursing procedures for reverse isolation. *Amer. J. Nurs.* 65:108, June 1965.

Schwartz, S., and others. The effect of bacterial suppression and reverse isolation on intensive cancer chemotherapy. *Clin. Res.* 13:48, Dec. 1965.

U.S. Public Health Service. *Isolation Techniques for Use in Hospitals* (PHS No. 2054). Washington, D.C.: U.S. Government Printing Office, 1970.

U.S. Public Health Service, Center for Disease Control. Isoniazid-associated hepatitis: Summary of the tuberculosis advisory committee and special consultants to the director, Center for Disease Control. *Morbidity and Mortality Weekly Report.* 23:97, Mar. 16, 1974.

STERILIZATION AND DISINFECTION

General texts

Becton, Dickinson Lectures on Sterilization, presented during the academic years 1957-1959 as part of the curriculum in bacteriology at Seton Hall, College of Medicine and Dentistry, Jersey City, N.J.

Disinfection of medical equipment. *Medical Letter on Drugs and Therapeutics.* 9(7) issue 215, Apr. 7, 1967.

Lawrence, C. A., and Block, S. S., editors. *Disinfection, Sterilization, and Preservation.* Philadelphia: Lea & Febiger, 1968.

Perkins, J. J. *Principles and Methods of Sterilization in Health Sciences.* 2nd ed. Springfield, Ill.: Charles C Thomas, 1969.

Spaulding, E. H. Recommendations for chemical disinfection of medical and surgical materials. Appendix B in *Environmental Aspects of the Hospital*, vol. 1, *Infection Control* (PHS No. 930-C-15). Washington, D.C.: U.S. Government Printing Office, 1966.

Sykes, G. *Disinfection and Sterilization.* 2nd ed. Philadelphia: J. B. Lippincott Co., 1965.

General references

Kelsey, J. C. The myth of surgical sterility. *Lancet.* 2:1301, Dec. 16, 1972.

Recommendations for the decontamination and maintenance of inhalation therapy equipment. Center for Disease Control. *National Nosocomial Infections Study Quarterly Report.* Third Quarter 1972, Aug. 1973.

Roberts, F. J., and others. Pasteurization of instruments. *Can. Med. Assn. J.* 101:30, July 12, 1969.

Rubbo, S. D., and Gardner, J. F. *A Review of Sterilization and Disinfection as Applied to Medical, Industrial, and Laboratory Practice.* 2nd ed. Chicago: Year Book Medical Publishers, 1965.

Standard, P. G., and others. Microbial penetration of muslin- and paper-wrapped sterile packs stored on open shelves and in closed cabinets. *Appl. Microbiol.* 22:432, Sept. 1971.

References to particular methods

Air disinfection with Ultra-violet irradiation: Its effect on illness among schoolchildren. *Med. Res-Council* (UK). 1954. Spec. reports, No. 2830 (By the Air Hygiene Committee).

Department of the Army, Chemical Corps. Maintenance of germicidal ultraviolet installations. *Technical Manual No. 2.* Fort Detrick, Md.: U.S. Army Biological Laboratories, 1963.

Doyle, J. E., and Ernst, R. R. Resistance of *Bacillus subtilis* var. *niger* spores occluded in water-soluble crystals to three sterilization agents. *Appl. Microbiol.* 15:726, July 1967.

Gilbert, G. L., and others. Effect of moisture on ethylene oxide sterilization. *Appl. Microbiol.* 12:496, Nov. 1964.

Jefferson, S., and others. Radiation sterilization of medical supplies. *Nuclear Engineering.* 9:284, Aug. 1964.

Matsumoto, T., and others. Safe standard of aeration for ethylene oxide sterilized supplies. *Arch. Surg.* 96:464, Mar. 1968.

National Tuberculosis and Respiratory Disease Association. *Infectiousness of Tuberculosis.* New York: NTA, 1967.

Postoperative wound infections: the influence of ultraviolet irradiation of the operating room and of various other factors (Report of an Ad Hoc Committee). *Ann. Surg.* Vol. 160, Special Supplement, Aug. 1964.

Proceedings of Symposium on Radiation Sterilization (Pub. No. ST-1-157). Vienna: International Atomic Energy Agency, 1966.

Riley, R. L., and Permutt, S. Room air disinfection by ultraviolet irradiation of upper air. *Arch. Environ. Health.* 22:208, Feb. 1971.

Skaliy, P. Ethylene oxide as a hospital sterilizing agent. *Hospitals, J.A.H.A.* 40:100, Nov. 16, 1967.

Warner, H. V. Untersuchungen uber die wirkung von ultraviolettstrahlen auf den keimgehalt der raumluften. [Investigation of the effect of ultraviolet rays on the germ content of room air.] *Schweiz. Med. Wschr.* 102:670, 1972.

Chapter 6

Special Problems

This chapter deals with special problems such as infected personnel, hazardous areas, and hazardous procedures. Effective infection control measures may be more difficult to achieve in these situations than in most, but they will be reflected in a lower nosocomial infection rate.

INFECTED PERSONNEL AND CARRIERS

Patients, staff, or visitors with active infection present a straightforward control problem. But symptomless carriers of pathogenic microorganisms present a highly complex problem in that protective measures and practicality may be in conflict. The etiologic agents of most acute communicable diseases are frequently harbored by clinically normal persons—those in the incubation period of the disease or those with trivial symptomology. Carrier rates for microorganisms causing nosocomial infection may be substantial. Rates of from 10 to 50 per cent have been recorded for both coagulase-positive staphylococci and group A streptococci among persons in the general population. Hospital personnel may be among these carriers.

Many authorities believe that symptomless carriers are frequently suffering from low-grade chronic infection with irregular episodes of minor symptoms. This belief tends to be supported by pathological findings commonly seen in chronic low-grade cholecystitis and cholangitis in typhoid carriers and in chronic inflammatory changes in the upper respiratory tract mucosa (or in lymphoid tissue) in persistent *Staphylococcus aureus* carriers. Although the distinction between a truly asymptomatic carrier and one with only minor symptoms may be important in individual instances, such a distinction is seldom of practical importance.

Routine Search for Carriers

In general, routine measures for identifying and dealing with carriers of pathogens are impractical. Experience has shown that routine screening is expensive and wasteful of personnel time and laboratory manpower. Moreover, such screening is usually unreliable and can give a false sense of security. In certain instances, however, state or local health departments may have mandatory legal requirements for screening examinations of food handlers.

Infection control committees in some hospitals have conducted routine screening examinations of certain groups working in particularly sensitive areas, such as surgical suites, obstetric suites, premature nurseries, and intensive care units. Such procedures are expensive and time consuming, and the potential benefit to be realized in the absence of a specific epidemiologic problem is so minor that this procedure is not recommended. Furthermore, in the absence of specific nosocomial infection in these areas, the removal of carriers identified during such screening examinations is not warranted as a general policy.

Specific Search for Carriers

Intensive searches, with rigorous investigative procedures, must be conducted for carriers who may be involved in an epidemic of a nosocomial infection. Suspects should be examined with due attention to their relationship to the outbreak.

Respiratory tract

Intensive searches for specific carrier states usually begin with respiratory tract examinations of suspected carriers. For diphtheria, the suspected carrier's nose and throat—tonsils and nasopharynx, including the back wall and upper surface of the soft palate—should be cultured.

When a search is made for carriers of hemolytic streptococci and meningococci, cultures should be obtained from tonsillar or nasopharyngeal lymphoid areas and from the throat.

Searches for carriers of staphylococci are usually made only in connection with an outbreak of disease. In such instances, carriers of the strain or strains causing the outbreak, as identified by phage type and antibiotic sensitivity pattern, should be sought among personnel. Epidemiologic characteristics of the outbreak should guide the screening. Unless there is exudate from chronic infection elsewhere in the upper respiratory tract, the anterior nares are the main site of bacterial colonization. Swabbing should be done from both nares.

The virulence of coagulase-positive staphylococci varies widely. Although in the past staphylococci of phage type 80/81 gained notoriety as a nosocomial pathogen, other phage types are well known to cause disease in hospitalized patients.

In assessing the significance of carriers of staphylococci among hospital personnel, careful consideration must be given the following facts:

- The nasal carrier rate among hospital personnel may vary from 10 to 70 per cent. The higher the carrier rate in personnel, the greater the potential for patient infection.
- About 15 per cent of adults seem to be incapable of supporting the growth of staphylococci in their nares, and up to 70 per cent are intermittent carriers. About 15 to 20 per cent are potentially permanent or at least long-term carriers. If a person is carrying coagulase-positive staphylococci in his nose, this does not necessarily mean that he is disseminating the organism. Even if he does, such dissemination does not necessarily result in disease among contacts.
- There is no reliable method by which nasal carriers of staphylococci can be cleared of their carrier state. At least 50 per cent of nasal carriers are also skin carriers. Systemically administered antibiotics usually suppress the carrier state only temporarily.

The evidence indicates that it is the permanent carrier of large numbers of staphylococci who is the greatest potential danger, particularly if there is associated evidence of disease such as furunculosis. A prolonged period of colonization of the nose by large numbers of staphylococci plus colonization of the skin, usually indicates a potential shedder or disseminator. If an organism is of the same phage type and antibiotic susceptibility pattern as that causing disease in patients with whom the individual has had contact, that person may then be implicated as the source.

Nasal cultures should be obtained from hospital personnel if clusters of cases of staphylococcal infection develop among patients directly under their care. If an individual is found to be carrying the same strain as that recovered from the patient's lesion, it still may not be possible to identify that person as the source of infection with certainty; he may have acquired the organism from the patient. The relative importance of any individual carrier in connection with an outbreak can be determined only by correlating culture findings with the epidemiologic evidence. Sequential cultures aid in identifying long-term, or chronic, staphylococcal carriage, a condition known to be associated with potential danger of transmission. Individuals identified as probable sources of infection should be removed from patient contact and given treatment in the hope of eliminating the carrier state.

No approach to treatment of the staphylococcal carrier state has been uniformly successful. Oral systemic antistaphylococcal therapy with cloxacillin or dicloxacillin usually suppresses, but does not eradicate, the carrier state. Bacitracin ointment or cream applied to the anterior nares three or four times daily for 10 to 14 days has sometimes been successful, but again, such therapy often merely suppresses rather than eradicates the carrier state. Close attention to personal hygiene, including the daily use of hexachlorophene-containing soap or detergent, may similarly be useful in reducing shedding and dissemination, but this should not be expected to achieve permanent eradication of the carrier state.

Group A beta-hemolytic streptococci occasionally are implicated in causing hospital-acquired streptococcal infection and are often traceable to personnel carriers. Personnel implicated epidemiologically as suspect should have cultures taken of the anterior nares, pharynx, and skin. Any beta-hemolytic streptococci isolated from such individuals should be studied by serologic grouping and typing procedures, in order to ascertain whether the strain recovered is identical to that isolated from patients. Occasional outbreaks have been traced to anal carriers of group A beta-hemolytic streptococci; this possibility should be considered.

Group B beta-hemolytic streptococci are increasingly recognized as a cause of serious disease in the neonatal period. The evidence suggests that the vast majority of such infections are acquired from the mother by the infant, although cross infection in the hospital may occur. The female reproductive tract appears to be a major reservoir of group B streptococci.

There is no evidence suggesting that hospital personnel are an important source of group B beta-hemolytic streptococci in the neonate, and screening of personnel for this organism is not recommended.

Intestinal tract

When epidemiologic circumstances indicate the need for a search for carriers of salmonellae, shigellae, or enteropathogenic *Escherichia coli,* culturing one stool or rectal swab from all suspected persons should be the first step. In this way, the offending carrier can often be identified promptly. The suspects may be cultured again on three successive days.

In searching for carriers of *Salmonella typhi,* preliminary screening of large groups by eliminating those who have no Vi agglutinins is of doubtful validity, since investigators have reported 10 to 30 per cent Vi-negative carriers. No one should be classified as a carrier or noncarrier on the basis of this serologic test alone.

Enteropathogenic *Escherichia coli* carriage by personnel may be important in the spread and persistence of outbreaks in the newborn nursery. A carrier may be identified by culture, if a case of disease is noted in the nursery.

In personnel suspected of transmitting amebiasis, at least one fresh stool should be examined in addition to a minimum of two specimens concentrated for amoebic cysts.

Hepatitis B

Because of the ability to identify hepatitis B antigen (HB Ag)—also called hepatitis-associated antigen (HAA) or Australia antigen—in the blood and the association of HB Ag with hepatitis B (serum hepatitis), problems arise concerning the management of hospital personnel found to be HB Ag positive.

If an HB Ag-positive person has symptoms of hepatitis, he should be treated and, if hospitalized, maintained under enteric precautions designed for patients with hepatitis B. If the patient is asymptomatic, testing for HB Ag should be repeated on a new serum specimen. If the positive result is confirmed, he should be further evaluated for the presence of hepatic disease. If none is found, the individual should be tested for HB Ag every three to six months until the test becomes negative. An individual who has acute hepatitis and whose blood is positive for HB Ag usually will revert to the negative status within six months.

Patient care personnel or staff found to be positive for HB Ag should be managed as described in Appendix D, page 182. (See also Appendix E, page 186.)

By far the most important route of transmission of HB Ag is parenteral, although some evidence from epidemiologic studies suggests occasional transmission by a nonparenteral route, such as airborne or oral. The precise mechanism and frequency of nonparenteral routes of transmission are currently under active study.

Management of Personnel Carriers

The mere identification of personnel carriers of a given pathogen does not, per se, require that they be treated or removed from patient care responsibilities. Data so derived must be interpreted in the light of epidemiologic investigation and must recognize that a given carrier may be just as easily the result of, rather than the cause of, hospital-acquired infection. If epidemiologic information implicates or makes highly suspect one or more persons found to be carriers of the pathogen causing hospital-acquired infection, then appropriate steps should be taken to deal with the problem.

In each case an attempt should be made to determine whether the individual has treatable abnormalities, such as chronic infection or contributory diseases such as allergic states or diabetes. Some carriers, for example, carriers of group A beta-hemolytic streptococci, can be expected to respond promptly to the administration of penicillin. Occasionally, penicillinase-producing staphylococci are also present and may inactivate the penicillin, so that group A streptococcal carriage may persist. In such instances, therapy with cloxacillin or dicloxacillin may prove useful.

The treatment of carriers of gastrointestinal tract pathogens, such as salmonella, shigella, and enteropathogenic *Escherichia coli,* is usually unnecessary, because most such carriers become negative spontaneously. Chemotherapy with drugs such as ampicillin, tetracycline, and neomycin often only suppresses rather than cures the carrier state. Such individuals can often best be managed by making them aware of their carrier status and reemphasizing the necessity of scrupulous personal hygiene. For chronic typhoid carriers, surgical intervention must be considered.

Many carrier states cannot be eradicated even with the best modern treatment. In some instances special preventive measures, such as retraining of personnel, reassignment to nonpatient contact duties, or palliative measures to reduce the number of organisms being carried or shed, can be designed to meet individual needs. Stubborn, permanent carriers of epidemic types of staphylococci are one of the most difficult problems, but it has been well demonstrated that even surgeons who are carriers may continue their activities safely if they take extra precautions, including careful masking, routine bathing, scrubbing with suitable disinfectants, thorough hand washing between patient contacts, and temporary suppression of nasal flora by using a suitable antibacterial ointment.

HAZARDOUS AREAS

Hazardous areas are those areas in which the services performed may predispose the recipient to the introduction of infection. Hazardous areas include blood banks, surgical suites, intensive care units, dialysis units, and newborn nurseries.

Blood Bank

Of all the biological products used in hospitals, blood is one of the most valuable. It is also a product frequently associated with hazards. Besides the well-known problems of proper matching, preservation, and adverse patient reactions, infectious microorganisms may be present in the blood at the time of collection or may be introduced during subsequent stages of processing.

Posttransfusion hepatitis is the most frequent exogenous nosocomial infection associated with the administration of blood. Although posttransfusion hepatitis remains the most serious infection transmissible by blood, it is now possible to detect the presence of HB Ag (hepatitis B antigen) in up to 50 per cent of potentially infective blood by using sensitive tests, such as the passive hemagglutination test or radioimmunoassay.

Not all posttransfusion hepatitis can be prevented by such donor screening, and the risk is therefore proportional to the number of donors. Donor populations of different geographic and socioeconomic backgrounds have various hepatitis carrier rates, the average in the United States being approximately one per cent. Blood obtained from blood banks using volunteer donors is known to be associated with the least risk of posttransfusion hepatitis, whereas blood obtained from commercial blood banks is known to carry a significantly higher risk. Products made from blood, except for gamma globulin and heat-treated fractions, also carry a risk related to the number and source of donors in the original pool. In addition to the considerable morbidity, the fatality rates in transfusion-associated hepatitis have exceeded 25 per cent in some studies. Further, an unknown proportion of patients develop evidence of chronic hepatic dysfunction, which may progress to cirrhosis.

Careful histories must be obtained from prospective donors, with particular reference to previous infectious disease. Prospective donors with any of the following findings should be rejected: fever; acute respiratory infection; dental surgery within the previous 72 hours; history of hepatitis or jaundice; history of close contact with a hepatitis patient within the previous six months; narcotic drug addiction or alcoholism; infectious skin disease at the venipuncture site; recent vaccination with a live virus (smallpox, measles, poliomyelitis, rubella, mumps, and yellow fever); and evidence of such diseases as malaria, measles, mumps, brucellosis, or syphilis. Travel or residence in an area where malaria is endemic requires a three-year symptom-free period after termination of chemoprophylaxis (six months' exclusion if chemoprophylaxis was not taken and the donor is asymptomatic). Donors who have had malaria or are immigrants or visitors from endemic areas may donate blood following three years' continuous residence in a nonendemic area. The American Red Cross should be contacted for its latest recommendations concerning plasma, plasma components, or fractions devoid of RBCs from prospective donors with malaria exposure. Any donor likely to have been responsible for a transmission of hepatitis in the past must not be permitted to donate again.

There rarely is adequate justification to transfuse a unit of blood that has not first been screened for the presence of HB Ag. Such screening should be routine in all blood banks.

As a general procedure, the skin must be carefully disinfected at the site of venipuncture, and the blood should be collected aseptically by means of a sterile, closed system. If a vented system is used, it must have a suitable bacterial air filter. In the preparation of plasma and packed cells, a closed system should be used and the processing should be done in a scrupulously clean room.

All personnel in the blood bank and in laboratories dealing with blood should be instructed in the techniques of blood handling, notably with reference to asepsis and to the proper use of equipment for collecting, processing, testing, and administering blood or blood products. All blood should be considered potentially infectious, and treated with the care due infectious material. All blood should be inspected before use; if its color or appearance is in any way abnormal, it should not be used but should be returned to the blood bank for study.

The safety precautions that should be observed by blood bank personnel are the same as those that apply in any hospital laboratory. Blood containing HB Ag and used HB Ag test materials should be autoclaved or incinerated.

In addition to hepatitis, syphilis and malaria may be transmitted by fresh whole blood. An infectious mononucleosis-like syndrome caused by cytomegalovirus has been increasingly recognized following blood transfusions. A false-positive tuberculin skin test may be transmitted by viable lymphocytes from a PPD-positive donor. The infectious complications of transfusions become all the more serious because they are not likely to be considered in the differential diagnosis.

Surgical Suite

The care of patients in the surgical suite requires the most stringent precautions for the prevention of infection. Not only are massive surgical and traumatic tissue wounds exposed for many hours to various equipment, supplies, personnel, and the air, but natural defenses are depressed by anesthetic drugs. Tubes and catheters are inserted into the nose, trachea, veins, arteries, and urinary bladder. Large and small foreign bodies are implanted in the tissue either temporarily or permanently. Many surgical patients also have acute and chronic illnesses that may increase susceptibility.

The quality of the operating room aseptic technique and cleanliness of the atmosphere, as well as the quality of the support given by other departments, is reflected in the postoperative infection rate.

The infection control committee provides an organizational framework for the collaboration of the departments involved in the activities related to infection control in the surgical suite. The committee relates to the surgical suite through its members, the chief of surgery or his representative, and the surgical nursing supervisor. As committee members, they advise on problems of infection following surgery and supply data on procedures, personnel, and so forth.

The chief of surgery and the surgical nursing supervisor are directly responsible for the suite's operation. The chief of surgery makes the policies, with appropriate administrative advice and consent, whereas the nursing supervisor implements them. The nursing supervisor is directly responsible for the nursing staff members and for such training as they may require. With all these duties, the nursing supervisor may spend more time within the operating suite than any other member of the hospital staff with executive responsibilities. In this unique position, the supervisor is best suited to carry out the policies of the chief of surgery and the infection control committee. Under the direction of the chief of surgery, the nursing supervisor must implement effective systems for personnel traffic, instrument handling, provision of expendable supplies such as solutions and laundry, general sterilization, and a regular cleaning schedule. Special provision must be made for infected or contaminated patients so that they can be handled safely without disrupting the schedule of the surgical department.

Asepsis

Sound practices of asepsis are fundamental to the prevention of infection within the surgical suite. Persons working in the suite must wear standard clean surgical costumes in lieu of their ordinary clothing. Surgical costumes should be designed for maximum skin coverage, because shedding of organisms from the skin is a potential source of contamination. It is undesirable to leave arms uncovered in the operating room. Persons who are not gowned should wear jackets or pullovers with long sleeves. Conductive shoes, to be worn only within clean areas, should also be available. Where laundry facilities permit, cloth boots with conductive soles should be used within the surgical suite. All head and facial hair should be completely covered. All personnel should wear double-thickness filter masks or efficient commercial deflection masks in the operating room and wherever sterile supplies are exposed. When masks become damp or wet after 40 to 45 minutes of use, they are no longer effective and must be changed. Surgical and nursing personnel should be allotted ample space outside the operating room for a complete change of clothing. If personnel wear surgical garb outside the surgical suite, they must change into fresh clothing on return.

Special clothing may be useful for certain types of cases: for example, double-lined gowns over a plastic apron are helpful in neurosurgery. This combination is generally useful in any surgery involving the use of considerable fluid, such as thoracic or genitourinary surgery, as the plastic prevents fluid contact between the wound areas and skin surfaces of personnel.

The surgical scrub is an essential part of personnel practice relating to infection prevention. A clearly visible schedule for this procedure should be posted on the wall next to the scrub sink, where a clock or timer should also be visible. Preparation for an adequate scrub should include at least nail cleaning with an orange stick and hand washing to remove surface oils. Generally speaking, personnel should keep their fingernails short and the skin of their hands and arms free from abrasion and infection. An infection on the hand, as well as furuncles on other parts of the body, are reasons for exclusion from surgery.

The patient's skin at the site of incision as well as a wide margin around it should be shaved and scrubbed in a manner similar to that used on the surgeon's hand. In elective surgery, all local or remote infection should be eradicated prior to the operation.

All skin of the patient should be covered either with an impervious drape or with sufficient thickness of pervious material to prevent fluid penetration during the procedure. This material, whether cloth, paper, or plastic, should also have sufficient strength to prevent gross mechanical penetration by instruments, hands, or equipment.

Since the nasopharynx of any person is a ready source of airborne organisms, all persons with upper respiratory infection should be excluded from work directly related to operating or the handling of sterile supplies, whenever possible. For similar reasons, and despite the wearing of masks, communication should be limited to essential conversation both over the wound and around exposed sterile supplies.

The asymptomatic nasal carrier of coagulase-positive staphylococci need not be excluded from the operating area unless he is a known spreader or unless an otherwise unexplained outbreak of coagulase-positive staphylococcal disease has occurred in operative wounds. In tracing the source of such disease it may be helpful to study phage typing, antibiograms of coagulase-positive staphylococci isolated from personnel, the environment, and other infections (see Management of Personnel Carriers, page 123).

Personnel should restrict movements to those required for the operation or its support. Excessive, unnecessary movements and conversation greatly increase shedding of skin organisms and movement of bacteria through the air. Normal traffic patterns for each type of infection should be analyzed and described so that personnel can be trained to use them. Establishing set procedures avoids waste motion and prevents excessive and inefficient activity. All aseptic procedures require study and analysis of the various wound requirements. Thus, practices for a thoracic exposure may differ from those required for cranial or pelvic procedures. Although the basic preparation of personnel (scrubbing, clothing, and so on) may be the same for all, the positions and traffic patterns are different. Certain wounds, such as those in the brain, require more vigorous precautions because of the tissue's greater vulnerability to infection.

Personnel practices

Effective infection control practices depend on the training and cooperation of all personnel concerned. Nursing and surgical personnel require extensive training. The cooperation, understanding, and concern of every senior surgeon are essential ingredients for success in the prevention of infection. In this regard, the chief of surgery and the nursing supervisor must assume roles as diplomats. A senior surgeon may cherish his own particular technique to the extent that he may be suspicious of a system threatening to change particular facets of it. Nonetheless, without loss of individual effectiveness, he may be tactfully brought to appreciate the need for rigid adherence to principles of infection control.

Visitors to the operating floor and adjacent spaces must be restricted. If the visit is essential, visitors must meet the clothing requirements of the surgical personnel. Only professionally concerned individuals who are free from infection may enter the actual suite under these conditions. Where an enclosed gallery with a separate ventilation system is available, such rigorous restrictions need not apply.

Equipment and instruments

Surgical furniture and other permanent equipment should be arranged to provide maximum efficiency for each type of case. All permanent equipment should be subject to regular cleaning by the operating room staff. This must include floors and walls, with particular attention to air ducts, sills, and other crevices. In addition to a daily cleaning of permanent equipment, all surfaces should be wiped twice daily, and any surface in contact with blood or other fluids should be scrubbed thoroughly after each procedure, as should the floor. Equipment such as television and other cameras and radiographic equipment used in operating rooms should be appropriately cleaned prior to their introduction into the operating room. Draping of such equipment is sometimes indicated.

All surgical instruments should be subject to thorough washing and preventive maintenance before sterilization. A dull knife or scissors, or a jagged rongeur, can contribute to wound morbidity by unnecessary tissue destruction. The packing of instruments and linen should be carried out with rigorous sterile precautions.

The most reliable method of sterilization available for each type of material should be used. The operating room supervisor must be certain that all requirements of cleaning, wrapping, packaging, and storage are met, whether the sterilizing process is carried out in the operating suite or elsewhere. The supervisor must also be satisfied that the physical factors necessary for sterilization of a given type of package by a given method have been met as outlined under Sterilization, page 95. The operating room supervisor must bear the final responsibility for use of adequate chemical and regular biologic indicators as described in the section on Sterilization and Disinfection, page 93.

As with surgical instruments, linen should be subject to preventive maintenance, and all packs returned from sterilization elsewhere should be examined for surface integrity. Regular examination of stored packs for integrity and dating is equally important. The surgical nursing supervisor should be aware of the handling and transportation systems for all incoming material and should monitor these systems for potential avenues of contamination.

Handling of anesthesia apparatus is described on page 143. Because it is an integral part of surgical equipment, the nursing supervisor should work closely with the anesthesiologist or anesthetist to establish consistent practices and high standards.

Expendable supplies are occasional sources of contamination. Each type of supply, such as sutures, solutions, wax, gauze, and so on, is handled directly or indirectly before it is brought to the operating room. The operating room supervisor must be satisfied that the materials arrive in the operating room sterile and that they are packaged in such a way that the personnel can introduce them into the operating field without contamination.

The infected patient

The contaminated or infected patient requires special procedures, which should be established and included in the surgical procedures manual. These should deal with personnel, furniture, equipment, and laundry, as well as with all areas used by the patient or contaminated by his secretions or fluids. Areas of cutaneous infection should be carefully covered with an inclusive dressing before the patient enters the operating room. Special, complete, and immediate cleaning of the operating room is essential. Laundry should be separated into different colored bags and should be collected in the contaminated room before bagging. No clothing or linen should leave the room unbagged. All instruments should be dropped in disinfectant solutions within the room; electronic equipment requires special treatment. All persons should scrub again after the case and after handling the infected material.

When there is a choice, operations on infected patients should be scheduled last in the course of the day's work. After completion of surgery, the room should be cleaned thoroughly. The ceiling and walls should be washed if there is gross contamination. Masks and caps should be worn until all the special cleaning has been completed.

Intensive Care Unit

The lifesaving potential of surgical, medical, or combined intensive care units has been demonstrated many times. Such units are usually crowded with equipment and personnel, and are necessarily extremely active. Patients in these units are seriously ill and severely compromised. Therefore, such patients are unusually susceptible to hospital-acquired infection, and even relatively small numbers of organisms of relatively low virulence can produce disastrous opportunistic infections.

The degree of crowding, the frequency with which emergency procedures such as tracheostomy, cardiac resuscitation, intravenous cutdowns, and so forth are performed, and the urgency that often accompanies these procedures combine to make intensive care units among the most highly contaminated areas in a hospital. Thus, these areas present an extremely high risk of nosocomial infection.

Several considerations are important in the prevention of nosocomial infection in intensive care units:
- Intensive care units should be designed to provide ample room for emergency care of individual patients. The efficiency of nursing care

may decrease appreciably if these areas are overcrowded with patients or equipment. Space should be allowed for necessary equipment, such as mechanical respirators, resuscitators, and monitors of temperature, pressure, and cardiac function. Because of the high rate of environmental contamination, good ventilation and strict daily cleaning regimes are necessary in these units. Hospital hygiene, particularly hand washing, can suffer under the pressures of intensive care. Therefore, sinks should be provided at several convenient locations throughout an intensive care area, so that personnel may conveniently wash their hands between patient contacts. A single sink, located at one end of a room, is not likely to be used by a nurse who is simultaneously giving care to acutely ill patients at the other end of the room.

- Staffing patterns should be established with care and, if possible, flexibility. Nursing requirements for intensive care units almost never can be predicted with accuracy from day to day, but nowhere can nursing care suffer as greatly as in an understaffed intensive care unit.

- Hazardous procedures such as tracheostomy, intravenous cutdowns, and the like are frequently employed in intensive care units. The precautions to be observed are described under Hazardous Procedures, page 141, but these precautions assume particular importance in intensive care units. Central venous catheters are often necessary in patients under intensive care; they should be inserted by using surgical aseptic technique and should be removed as soon as practicable. Monitoring equipment requiring parenterally inserted probes or leads similarly demands careful aseptic care during insertion and maintenance.

- Intensive care units should not be used for isolation. The use of intensive care units has helped in achieving a significant improvement in hospital care of many seriously ill patients, as well as a more efficient use of nursing personnel. On the other hand, intensive care units are also ideal locations for cross infection when infected patients are permitted in these units. Infected patients and patients requiring isolation techniques should not be permitted in intensive care units unless special arrangements are made to achieve effective isolation.

- It is neither feasible nor humane to deny visiting privileges to acutely ill patients in intensive care units. It is feasible and often necessary, however, to limit visiting to a specified length of time and to limit the total number of visitors to a level consistent with the efficient operation of the intensive care unit.

- Hand washing between patient contacts remains the single most important method of control of cross infection in hospitals and assumes critical importance in this high-risk area.

Dialysis Unit

All the information pertaining to intensive care units applies with equal validity to dialysis units. However, an unusual frequency of cases and outbreaks of hepatitis A and B have occurred among patients and personnel in dialysis units, so the following comments apply particularly to this problem.

Several considerations form a basis on which recommendations can be made. Dialysis patients who receive frequent transfusions seem to have the highest risk of developing hepatitis A or B. In addition, hepatitis among dialysis patients is frequently asymptomatic; however, these asymptomatic patients may be implicated in the spread of hepatitis. Periodic screening of chronic dialysis patients for HB Ag is useful to detect asymptomatic patient carriers. Not all dialysis-associated hepatitis patients, however, are positive for HB Ag.

Dialysis nurses frequently have manual contact with blood. Although they are exposed to hepatitis B from accidental needle punctures and exposure to blood, not all nurses who develop hepatitis can recall this type of injury. Although the principal problem in dialysis units has been parenteral transmission of hepatitis B, there is evidence that nonparenteral transmission of hepatitis B may occur, as well as transmission of hepatitis A by either route.

The following recommendations can be expected to reduce the risk of hepatitis among the staff of dialysis units:
- Staff should avoid using needles whenever possible in order to minimize the chance of autoinoculation with infective blood. Rather, tubing that permits removal of blood by stopcock control should be used. If needles must be used, they should be used only with great care. Instead of recapping needles, they should be deposited uncapped into a disposable plastic bottle kept at each bedside. When full, the bottle may be capped and subsequently autoclaved or incinerated. Consideration may be given to a system for identifying known positive HB Ag patients.
- The chances of ingesting infective blood may be minimized by scrupulous attention to handwashing habits and by wearing disposable gloves while handling shunts, drawing blood, dismantling equipment, removing patient excreta, and so forth. In addition, staff personnel

should not be allowed to keep food, eat, or smoke in the dialysis area. Any habit of personal hygiene involving oral contact, for example, nail biting or putting pencils in mouth, must be avoided. Other types of infection may present hazards and require consideration.
- As in intensive care units, handwashing areas should be easily accessible. Separate toilet facilities should be made available for patients and staff personnel. Dialysis equipment should be disposable whenever possible; permanent equipment such as the dialysis tanks should be cleansed and decontaminated daily to remove organic material (see below). Tanks should be thoroughly dried overnight to avoid growth of aerobic gram-negative bacilli such as pseudomonas or flavobacteria in moist areas. Shunt sites should be inspected for evidence of infection before each dialysis.
- Because patients undergoing dialysis for acute renal failure are much less likely to be carriers of HB Ag than patients on chronic dialysis, these two groups of patients should be kept physically separate and preferably should be cared for by separate nursing staffs.

Much of the hepatitis occurring in dialysis units appears to be associated with HB Ag, against which immune serum globulin has not proven beneficial. However, there is evidence that some outbreaks of hepatitis have been caused by the agent of infectious hepatitis (hepatitis A), against which immune serum globulin is known to be effective. If the precise etiologic diagnosis is unknown, or if infectious hepatitis is suspected, immune serum globulin should be given in a dose of 0.01 milliliter per pound of body weight to personnel following accidental parenteral or oral exposure. The use of immune serum globulin on a routine basis, however, is not recommended for personnel working in dialysis units.

The following directions* are suggested for cleaning dialysis machines:
1. Put on gloves.
2. Remove and discard coil and lines.
3. Rinse the sides of the tank and the compartment with cold tap water via hose connected to main line.
4. Drain.
5. Half fill the tank with water; add a solution of 5.25 per cent of sodium hypochlorite. Turn on dialysate pump, and completely open flow meter.
6. Fill compartment with water and one-fourth cup of bleach. Turn on recirculating pump.

---

*Provided by George E. Schreiner, M.D., professor of medicine, Georgetown University, for use in a 10-gallon machine.

7. With a damp towel, wipe blood pump and so forth, to remove dialysate and blood.
8. After seven minutes, drain, rinse with tap water, and drain again.
9. Half fill the tank with water, turn on dialysate pump, completely open flow meter, fill compartment with water, turn on recirculating pump.
10. After five minutes, check with Hemastix for presence of bleach. If positive, repeat rinse; if negative, drain and dry machine.
11. Open screw cap at side of reservoir tank to drain completely, and replace cap.

Newborn Nursery

The newborn infant quickly acquires bacterial flora from other individuals and from its environment. The mother, hospital personnel and equipment, and other infants in the nursery contribute to this acculturation. Because many microorganisms are potentially pathogenic for the newborn, measures should be taken to protect the infant from undue microbial exposure. This is necessary because the infant possesses relatively poor immunological mechanisms and lacks the ability to cope with certain pathogenic microorganisms. He is particularly susceptible to those organisms responsible for many enteric, respiratory, and cutaneous infections. Passive immunity transmitted from the mother is helpful against some microorganisms.

Nursery design

Because of the infant's susceptibility, nurseries should be planned with special care. Nurseries for newborn and premature infants should be near the obstetrical service, preferably on the same floor, and close to the delivery rooms. These nurseries should be separated from the main traffic flow of the hospital, and they must not be near areas where patients with communicable diseases are treated. The nurseries should be located to minimize travel from the nursery to the mother's room. Care should be taken to avoid placing linen chutes, refuse chutes, and the like within or near the nursery.

No precise recommendations can be given as to bassinet space requirements needed to minimize the transfer of infection. Many states now require a minimum of 24 square feet. When planning new nurseries, it is suggested that 30 square feet be allowed per bassinet in order to permit adequate working space and to minimize the possibility of transfer of infection.

Because airborne microorganisms may be important in the transmission of certain types of infection, the nursery ventilation system should provide frequent changes of room air. A minimum of 12 changes per hour should be adequate. The air system should provide a slight positive pressure in order to reduce cross currents from the corridor. Air from other areas in the hospital must not be circulated through the nurseries.

Cohort plan

The cohort plan is the generally preferred method of nursery management for normal newborn infants. This plan is designed to keep infants born during the same interval (no more than 48 hours) in the same nursery. By this method individual nursery units are filled and emptied at definite intervals and the transfer of potentially hazardous infections is limited to infants of one graduating class. The cohort plan also prevents older infants from transferring endemic infection between successive generations of infants. The factor of nontransference is particularly important in reducing the chances of staphylococcal infection, as this infection often is not recognized until days or even weeks after the infant has been discharged from the hospital.

After the infants of each cohort have been discharged, the nursery should be thoroughly cleaned and its equipment decontaminated before more infants are admitted. Although larger nurseries (up to eight infants) are convenient in large hospitals, in small hospitals it may be necessary to use nurseries as small as four bassinets, with one nurse in charge of two units, in order to maintain the cohort plan of operation.

No matter how many beds are available for postpartum care, individual nursery units should not accommodate more than eight bassinets. Even if the cohort plan is not adopted, the use of small nurseries tends to confine the transfer of microorganisms to small groups of infants, not large groups as happens in large nursery units. Large nurseries are also much less flexible in the control of nursery epidemics. Small nursery units may be designed in pairs, each nursery accommodating from four to eight infants and sharing a common work area.

Special units

In addition to the regular units, four different types of special units are necessary for optimal operation of the nursery. Small hospitals with low nursery census or adequate referral facilities may modify such standards; advance agreement may be required from local and/or state health authorities.

- A suspect nursery should be provided for infants who may be harboring a potentially serious infectious agent. For example, infants born of mothers suspected of harboring or incubating an infectious disease should be admitted to this unit. It also should be used for the care of infants who have undergone circumcision. Although suspect nursery units have been used for the admission of infants born outside the hospital delivery room or outside the hospital, this practice is currently being abandoned in many nurseries. The unit should be separate but conveniently located in relation to the newborn nursery; the work area should not be shared with that of the normal nursery.

  If the suspicion of infection is not confirmed after an appropriate interval of observation, the infant may be returned to the normal or special care nurseries unless he has been exposed to an infant with proven infection.

- An isolation unit is also essential for the care of infants after a definite diagnosis of infection has been made. This unit should be physically separate from the main and suspect nurseries, and it must not share facilities with other nursery units. The isolation unit and its work area must be properly washed or otherwise decontaminated prior to transfer of infants into the unit. Cleaning routines must be established.

- A nursery for the care of high-risk infants should be available. Infants admitted to this unit include premature and low-birth-weight infants, term infants requiring special observation, and those infants recovering from surgical procedures performed in the newborn period. This unit should be located in the same general area as the other nurseries, but it must be separate with respect to both personnel and facilities. Infants graduating from this nursery should not be transferred to the regular nursery after residence in the high-risk unit but may be admitted to the pediatric unit if they cannot be discharged to their homes. Because of the extended period of stay in the high-risk nursery, sometimes for as much as several months, the cohort system described for the normal newborn infant is not possible. Individual incubators have reduced the need for observation units and cohort plans in this type of nursery. Therefore, larger rooms have been found to be more functional and not associated with increased risk. Each bassinet or incubator within the larger rooms should have its own equipment, including equipment for baths and all necessary daily care. The incubators and bassinets may be arranged around the sides of the room, with a work area for charting and so forth, but infant care should not be done in the center. It is convenient to use floor markers to delineate areas in order to control bassinet placement, traffic patterns, and so forth.

- An observation nursery located close to the delivery suite to which the infant is transferred immediately after delivery for the first few hours of life is recommended. The infant is kept here until his temperature is stable and his status can be determined. He then can be transferred to the normal nurseries or the special care areas, as appropriate. Infants born outside the hospital and who appear normal may be admitted to this nursery before being transferred to the normal nurseries. In smaller hospitals, the admitting cohort nursery may also serve as the observation nursery.

Procedures

Procedures in the nursery should be standardized and should follow the recommendations of both the infection control committee and the health department. It should be emphasized again that of all the procedures available, hand washing is the single most important factor. Hand washing before touching each infant and his individual equipment for any reason must be standardized and rigorously enforced. Nursery procedures should be evaluated to be certain that no common bathing tables or common items of equipment are utilized, as sharing equipment between infants has been shown to transmit infection readily, despite attempts at decontamination.

Personnel regularly assigned to the nursery are not required to wear gowns over the scrub suit or similar dress worn in the nursery, nor are they required to wear masks. In the past, transient personnel, such as physicians and maintenance workers, have been required to scrub and don mask and gown prior to entering the nursery, but recent data suggest that the requirements are probably unnecessary except prior to direct contact with infants.

The umbilical cord must be clamped or tied with a sterile material. The stump should be observed daily for signs of inflammation. Subsequent care includes daily applications of 70 per cent alcohol or a suitable antibacterial substance in order to lessen the chances of infection.

A one per cent aqueous solution of silver nitrate prepared in individual ampules should be applied to the conjunctivae at birth. The eyes should be observed for evidence of infection while the infant remains in the nursery. Antibiotic agents may be used if approved by the health authorities and by the hospital staff. It is uncertain at the present time whether penicillin is suitable as a prophylactic agent, because sensitization may be induced in some infants.

Daily hexachlorophene baths are no longer recommended as a routine procedure. However, during periods of increased incidence of staphylococcal disease and when other control measures have been unsuccessful, a daily hexachlorophene bath may be used for two days for term infants if followed by careful rinsing. Daily application of antimicrobial ointment or antimicrobial dyes to the umbilical cord stump has also been useful in inhibiting bacterial colonization of infants during outbreaks of staphylococcal disease.

Increased attention to hand washing by personnel is required, and procedures must be reviewed to identify those factors favoring transfer of infection between infants. Dry skin care has been found to be satisfactory in many nurseries. Also, a search for carriers among personnel may be indicated.

The housekeeping personnel should be trained in proper sanitizing procedures; if infants are present in the nursery, housekeepers may wear suitable masks and gown while working, but many nurseries have abandoned this procedure during recent years.

Floor equipment and visibly soiled walls should be washed or wet-mopped thoroughly at the time of discharge of each cohort of infants. If the cohort plan is not used, daily cleaning routines should be accomplished at a time when the infants are out of the nursery, in order to minimize personnel contact with infants. At least every three months, and preferably more frequently, intensive cleaning of the nursery and all equipment must be done, and infants must be temporarily transferred to another area if necessary.

All incubators and bassinets must be washed and decontaminated between occupancy. After removal of bedding and attachments, a thorough washing with antiseptic detergent solution can reduce the risks of infection. Disposable bassinets may reduce cleaning costs. Some disposable bassinet units may be taken home on discharge of the infant and are inexpensive and practical for most nurseries.

Nursery equipment should be individualized for each nursery unit insofar as possible. Special care should be taken regarding the proper sterilization of nebulizers containing water, as these may harbor microorganisms such as pseudomonas. Formulas must be prepared and stored in accordance with standard procedures such as those stated in the American Hospital Association's manual *Procedures and Layout for the Infant Formula Room* and also those stated in state and local health department regulations.

Health records

The hospital should establish and maintain policies about the health of nursery personnel. Policies should require the accurate reporting of all employee illnesses. Accurate health records of all employees must be kept, with particular attention being paid to the prompt reporting of cutaneous lesions and of gastrointestinal and respiratory complaints.

Persons with active infections, after examination by a physician, should be excluded promptly from the nursery and the formula room and from contact with other infants and their mothers. If they cannot assume duties elsewhere in the hospital, time off with compensation should be provided. Paid time off helps to ensure adequate reporting of illnesses. Individual health reports and examinations can be used to prevent persons with recurrent furunculosis from being assigned to the nursery.

Suitable dressing rooms and locker facilities should be available close to the nursery where the nurses can change from street clothes to scrub suits or other appropriate nursery dress. The hospital should also provide preassignment physical examinations, including chest x-rays, for all nursery personnel.

Problems of infection

In view of the importance of prompt recognition and isolation of infants with infection, nursery nurses must be authorized to transfer any infant to an observation nursery when there is suspicion of infection. They should also be authorized to obtain stool or other appropriate cultures at the time of transfer. Infants should be retained in the observation unit for at least 24 hours, after which they may, on order of the attending physician, be returned to the routine nursery. If definite infectious disease has appeared among other infants in the observation unit while the infant in question is in residence, he and other infants must remain there or be transferred to the isolation nursery until discharged from the hospital. These infants must not be returned to the main nursery.

All infections occurring in the nursery should be reported to the infection control committee. If more than a single case of serious infectious disease appears in the nursery within a week, the fact should be reported promptly to the local health department. Immediate transfer of the infected infant or infants should be made to the isolation unit, and the nursery in which the infection was identified must be closed to further admissions until all infants present have been discharged. Careful washing of the unit and disinfection of all equipment must then be carried out.

In the event of multiple infections, emergency facilities with separate staff and equipment must be established in another area of the hospital. An alternative is for each infant to be cared for in the individual mother's room, with 24-hour rooming-in.

A full investigation of multiple infections by the infection control committee is mandatory, and the assistance of the local health department may be indicated. Careful attention should be directed to discovering the source and mechanism of infection, to prevent future outbreaks. Depending upon the type of infection and the probable methods of transfer, investigation should also cover possible roles of personnel, patients, and errors in technique or procedures in the formula room or formula service, the laundry, and the sterilizing equipment, as well as the facilities within the nursery. After the mechanisms and the etiologic agent have been identified and the epidemic controlled, careful washing of the nursery and decontamination of all equipment must be done prior to reopening the unit for the admission of new patients. The nursery staff members should be appropriately examined and tested prior to reassignment to the cleaned and reopened unit, because they may be latent carriers of the microorganisms responsible for the epidemic.

HAZARDOUS PROCEDURES

Hazardous procedures are performed not only in special service areas—the surgical suite, for example—but often at the bedside as well. These procedures may depress natural resistance mechanisms; they may also introduce pathogenic microorganisms into patients' systems. Special precautions are necessary, therefore, to prevent the inception of infection during anesthesia, inhalation therapy, tracheostomy, surgical dressing, and catheterization.

Anesthesia

The administration of anesthesia as a part of a surgical procedure is essentially an operating room function; it must be viewed as coming under the general regulations for the operating theater. However, some types of anesthesia are administered to hospitalized or ambulatory patients in other parts of the hospital.

The relationships of anesthesia to the hazards of nosocomial infection are complicated and varied. Pneumonia is always a possible complication of anesthesia. Predisposing factors may include suppression of respiration, interference with cough and tracheal cleansing, and irritative injury or edema of the bronchi and lungs. Contamination of anesthesia equipment may favor respiratory infection by pseudomonas or other bacteria.

In guarding against such hazards the following precautions are recommended. First, anesthetists and their assistants must dress in clean operating room clothing, with special operation room shoes or boot covers. Hands and forearms must be scrubbed. Anesthetists or assistants with any kind of active infection, particularly respiratory or cutaneous infection, must not enter the operating rooms. In operating rooms, caps and masks must be worn. Masks should be changed between cases or when they become wet. Only in exceptional circumstances should staff go from one operating room to another without rescrubbing and redressing; an anesthetist going to another room only to supervise the work of an assistant would represent such an exception.

When an anesthetist is to assist directly with an operation, is to handle surgical instruments, or is to give regional or spinal injections, he must perform the standard surgical hand scrub and use sterile gloves. Regardless of the type of anesthesia to be used, a protective screen must be placed between the patient's face and the operative site before skin preparation is finished. When an infected patient is undergoing surgery, the anesthetist must designate special infection control procedures at the time of the preoperative visit. The anesthetist must also arrange for specialized recovery room care in order to protect other patients.

Special procedures

Anesthesia must be considered as a minor surgical procedure demanding such precautions as preliminary hand scrubbing, standard preparations of the patient's skin (scrub, iodine, and alcohol), and the wearing of gloves.

During anesthesia, measures directed against cross contamination must be practiced. The difficulties in cleaning endoscopic and inhalation therapy equipment probably account for the disregard of adequate decontamination procedures for such equipment after use. However, the hazards inherent in the use of these kinds of equipment with infants are well known. In dealing with specific infections of high virulence, careful efforts to sterilize the equipment must be made. Demonstrated hazards and increased susceptibility of many patients to infection suggest that stricter attention should be paid to decontamination of equipment.

The need for special processing of endoscopic, anesthesia, and inhalation therapy equipment is based on the following facts. Equipment coming into direct contact with the upper respiratory tract is invariably contaminated with microorganisms present in respiratory secretions. Other components of equipment at a distance from the patient also tend to become contaminated with airborne microorganisms. The moist environment in all components of the equipment tends to support the growth of microorganisms, whether from the air, previous patients, or the tap water used in washing the equipment.

Care of equipment

The care of equipment and supplies, apart from the drawing of sterile disposables or standard sets from central supply, is sometimes a responsibility of the department of anesthesia. In the training of personnel and in the organizing of the work, a clear distinction should be made between complete sterility—the attempt to eliminate all living microorganisms—and disinfection or decontamination—the effort to destroy usual nonspore-forming microorganisms.

Of the many routine procedures necessary in the practice of anesthesiology, the following are suggested. After each use, all surfaces of anesthesia machines and tables should be wiped with a cloth soaked in a 2 per cent solution of chlorophenol or in a 450 parts per million iodophor solution. The machines should be kept covered with a clean cloth until put into use again. At the end of each day, machines, tables, and trolleys should be thoroughly washed with the same solution and removable parts should be disassembled for complete cleaning. After use with patients known to be infected, the machines and their parts should be cleaned and disinfected thoroughly.

There is conflicting evidence of the self-cleaning potentials of soda lime containers. Most of them can be used to the end of their efficiency without cleaning. When the soda lime needs to be renewed, or when it has been used on an infected patient, the canister should be emptied and washed thoroughly with a disinfectant. Separate connectors from the containers may be autoclaved. Machines having bayonet-type or slip-on attachments for containers are preferable, as ease of removal facilitates cleaning. Unidirectional valves should be treated in the same way as containers.

Two sets of corrugated rubber tubing should be allotted to each machine. The used set should be washed out with a disinfectant solution for 10 minutes and hung to drain while the clean set is substituted. The most practical cleaning method is to use a container large enough to support the tubing in an upright position, in order to avoid air pockets. An iodophor solution is recommended. A 0.25 per cent solution of acetic acid can also be used. The tubing can be autoclaved or, for special reasons, may be treated with ethylene oxide.

Y-connectors can be treated together with the corrugated tubing, or they can be washed separately with activated glutaraldehyde, iodophor solution, or a 0.25 per cent solution of acetic acid. Unidirectional valves that are mounted on the Y-connectors should be taken apart and treated as the Y-connectors are after each use.

Endotracheal connectors should be autoclaved after each use. Endotracheal tubes of metallized rubber should be autoclaved; if plastic, they can be sterilized with ethylene oxide, or they can be immersed for 10 minutes in activated glutaraldehyde and followed by thorough rinsing in sterile water.

Rebreathing bags should be rinsed with water and then filled with an iodophor solution or a 0.25 per cent acetic acid solution. The bag should be left lying flat for 10 minutes to give the residue of the disinfectant time to act. Finally, the bag should be rinsed thoroughly.

Oropharyngeal and nasopharyngeal tubes should be autoclaved. After being cleaned, laryngoscope blades should be soaked in activated glutaraldehyde or iodophor solution for 10 minutes.

If face masks are of solid rubber, they should be autoclaved. If the mask has an air-filled cushion, it should be in a single piece with a solid base and should have a bung that can be removed before autoclaving. Flash autoclaving—three minutes at 132°C. (270°F.)—is adequate. Because all types of chemical disinfection seem to cause contact dermatitis in considerable numbers of individuals, no particular procedure can be recommended.

Inhalation Therapy

Inhalation therapy and the use of respirators are often under the supervision of the anesthesiology department, but may also be the responsibility of a specialized cardiorespiratory or pulmonary service or of an internal medicine service. Although there is no need to observe operating room standards of gowning and masking of personnel, the necessity for rigorous decontamination and daily care of all equipment is the same for inhalation therapy as it is for anesthesia.

A wide variety of equipment is available for the administration of oxygen and of other gases and aerosols, including various types of tents, masks, and atomizers. In large hospitals the main difficulty lies in the organization of a reliable servicing facility. As a rule, centralized care of such equipment allows the least number of lapses, or errors, and provides for the most efficient methods of sterilization. However, personnel in various types of intensive care units using such equipment sometimes prefer to care for their own equipment or to arrange to have the central care facility placed next to the intensive care unit.

The importance of washing and disinfection of all equipment used for a patient has been described. In some hospitals there may be a considerable use of mobile suction apparatus and, when frequent suctions are required on a patient, the same catheter is used repeatedly. The cleaning and servicing of such suction machines is best done by those looking after the gas therapy and aerosol equipment. Catheters for reuse on such suction machines should be kept in a reservoir containing a disinfectant solution such as one per cent activated glutaraldehyde, changed daily; catheters must be rinsed in sterile water or saline solution before reuse.

For respirators and infant incubators, routine use varies from one hospital to another, and arrangements for care vary accordingly. Where there are a number of these instruments always in use, servicing and cleaning should be centralized in the department responsible for inhalation therapy. The maintenance of incubators or other equipment for newborn and premature infants is supervised as a rule by the nursery staff. For increased efficiency, however, the major cleaning and proper care of the humidification apparatus may be assigned to a centralized inhalation therapy department. For all apparatus, the same principles apply: washing and disinfecting must be done after each use, and the disinfectants should be selected and tested under the supervision of the infection control committee.

As pointed out by Pierce and Sanford, humidifiers that bubble a stream of gas through water generally do not produce significant aerosols and thus do not convey bacteria in the effluent gas. Reasonable measures to reduce the risk of contamination include: (1) fresh tubing should be supplied for each patient; (2) a single humidifier sterilized by ethylene oxide, autoclaving, or soaking in phenolic disinfectant should be furnished each patient who requires it; and (3) the residual liquid in the bottom of the humidifier should be discarded before the humidifier is refilled. Oxygen tents, nursery isolettes, and rapid-flow humidifiers used with ventilators all require this type of care.

Nebulizers constitute the greatest hazard in inhalation therapy. The following steps should be taken to minimize contamination: (1) All inside surfaces of the nebulizer should be handled in a sterile manner. (2) Only sterile solutions should be put into the nebulizer. (3) Only sterile water should be used. (4) Liquid condensate in the tubing between the nebulizer and the patient should never be drained back into the nebulizer jar, as it may be contaminated with bacteria-laden secretions from the patient. (5) When the reservoir jar is to be filled, the residual solution should be discarded and the jar should be rinsed with tap water. (6) Daily decontamination of the equipment should include gas sterilization with ethylene oxide, autoclaving, or decontamination with 0.25 per cent acetic acid; for most "all-purpose" types of nebulizers, daily aerosolization of 0.25 per cent acetic acid through the nebulizer for 10 minutes at the bedside is satisfactory and effective.

Gas-driven nebulizers utilizing the Venturi principle, but also containing large surface baffles, spinning-disc nebulizers, and ultrasonic nebulizers, cannot be decontaminated by acetic acid. They must be sterilized by autoclaving or by ethylene oxide. Either process must be carried out at least once daily.

Proper sterilization of endoscopic and bronchoscopic instruments after use should prevent the transmission of infection from one patient to other patients or to personnel.

Tracheostomy

Because a tracheostomy provides an airway directly into the lungs through which suctioning can be accomplished, this procedure may also afford access for many potentially pathogenic microorganisms. Persons caring for patients with tracheostomies must have special training in techniques required to lessen the dangers of infection. The discussion of equipment, procedures, and specific precautions that follows is intended as a guide and should be modified by the infection control committee and appropriate clinical departments to provide detailed procedures in accordance with local resources and requirements.

Required equipment includes: a suction machine or proper wall outlet; catheters of appropriate sizes, with a Y-tube connection to the suction machine; a collection bottle with one inch of water or a disinfectant in the base to facilitate cleaning; and an antibacterial solution (see Table 8, page 106).

Infection control relating to tracheostomies is mainly concerned with the suctioning procedure. In this procedure, mucus must be removed from the lower respiratory tract on prescription, on indications of patient distress, or on the appearance of mucus at the tube opening. The following steps should be taken in the tracheostomy suctioning procedure:
- Wash hands with soap or antibacterial detergent solution.
- Remove inner cannula, if necessary, and start the suction machine.
- Turn patient's head to one side and instill into the tube opening at least three medicine dropperfulls of sterile normal saline solution. This often aids in the removal of secretion.
- Insert catheter into the tracheostomy tube, and pass it to its full extent until the tracheal bifurcation is reached.

- Remove the catheter by placing a thumb on the Y-tube, allowing suctioning to continue and rotating the catheter slowly while withdrawing it.
- Repeat the procedure with the patient's head turned to opposite side.
- Flush the catheter with water after it has been withdrawn; then wipe it with sterile tissue, and replace it in the antiseptic solution until it is needed again.
- Wash hands.

A sterile soft rubber catheter, with two or more holes near the tip, should be used. The catheter should be connected to the proper Y-tube adapter without handling or contaminating the tip. An open-end Y-tube should connect the catheter to the suction equipment. This permits finger control for delivering intermitten suction during withdrawal of the tube, to avoid unnecessary trauma. Catheters must be changed at least every 24 hours or whenever contamination is suspected. They should be stored in an antiseptic solution, renewed, and maintained as already described.

The tracheostomy tube should be changed as necessary or at not less than one-week intervals; changes must be made by a physician. The inner cannula should be removed at least every eight hours and cleaned carefully by being washed in activated glutaraldehyde or phenolic compound. The interior should be cleaned with sterile pipe cleaners and the tube carefully rinsed with sterile water. At least twice daily the skin around the tube should be cleaned thoroughly with a standard bland antibacterial detergent solution. The nose and mouth should be suctioned with care as necessary; never should a catheter be used that will subsequently be used in the tracheostomy.

Warm humidification of the air entering the tracheostomy is essential, as the normal moistening function of the upper respiratory tract has been lost. Equipment should deliver a fine droplet mist; it should be maintained in accordance with principles outlined previously. Antibiotic prophylaxis as a routine procedure in tracheostomy is not recommended. Unless there is an emergency situation, appropriate cultures should be obtained if the material removed from the tracheostomy is discolored, bloody, or foul. Based on the specific sensitivities of the microorganisms identified, appropriate antibiotic therapy should be used if indicated. In an emergency, direct gram stains of the exudate are helpful in guiding therapy until cultures can be obtained.

In persons with tracheostomies, pseudomonal or staphylococcal infection and superinfection often create serious problems in therapy. It is apparent from various studies that the staff and patients frequently exchange microorganisms from tracheostomy wounds and from lower respiratory tract infections in these patients. Tracheostomies have been a source of herpes and streptococcal infections in the fingers of nurse attendants. Moreover, staphylococcal and streptococcal infections of the tracheostomy wound have developed when staff members with skin infections have been in attendance. Appropriate measures associated with the care of the catheter and of the skin around the tracheostomy must be taken. Handwashing procedures are particularly important in helping to prevent transfer of infection.

Surgical Dressing

Dressing a wound is a surgical procedure and should be carried out with the precision and care of an operative technique. Thus, each dressing should be applied with sterile precautions as well as with carefully planned methodology.

The anatomical location and surgical characteristics of each wound determine the shape, weight, consistency, and size of the dressing. Moreover, patient comfort usually dictates some characteristics of each dressing. Pressure, adhesive tension, bulk, and surface can usually be modified for comfort without sacrificing aseptic integrity or maintenance of the wound environment.

Aseptic integrity and maintenance of external wound environment are two principal objectives of every dressing. All materials used should be sterile and should be available in packages or containers at the dressing site. Special drugs may be required, irrigation solutions may be necessary, or surgical instruments may be needed in the dressing procedure. Therefore a set of dressing instruments should be available in a sterile pack, and the drugs and solutions ordinarily used by the attending staff should be accessible in containers that allow sterile dispensation.

Dressings can be applied directly to the patient either from a bedside cart or in a room modified or designed for the purpose. The same room can be used as a minor surgical operating room. There is no question that centralization of surgical functions in a ward unit provides a greater consistency of technique.

Dressings removed from the patient must be regarded as contaminated whether or not clinical evidence of infection is present. A suitable closed container must be available on the dressing cart for disposal of used dressings.

The frequency of dressing is a matter for surgical judgment. Each procedure should be regarded as a surgical operation, for the nature of the dressing technique may determine the biological course of the wound. Careful attention must be given to procedure and to training personnel for this important duty.

The personnel who change dressings require surgical training. Ideally, this training should be available to all nursing staff, but actually it may be necessary to train relatively few individuals in each nursing unit. Although dressings are usually applied by the day shifts, someone on night shifts must be skilled in the application. Usually, a surgeon and one nurse can successfully accomplish the necessary tasks. In so doing, they should wear masks and gloves. Hands should be washed before and after this procedure (see Table 10, below).

Catheterization

A large number and variety of catheters are employed in hospitals. The two kinds most often associated with serious infection in patients are urinary and venous catheters. The proper handling of all catheters, however, is essential for prevention of nosocomial infection. The use of disposable single-use catheters is recommended whenever possible.

Urinary catheters

Catheterization of the urinary tract is the greatest single cause of nosocomial urinary tract infection; the procedure should be done only when

Table 10
DRESSING TECHNIQUES

	Special	Standard
Hand washing, before	Necessary	Necessary
Gloves (2 sets)*	Necessary	Not necessary
Gown[†]	Necessary	Not necessary
Mask	Necessary	Not necessary
Sterile equipment	Necessary	Necessary
Double-bag technique for soiled dressings and equipment	Necessary	Necessary
No-touch technique	Necessary	Necessary
Hand washing, terminal	Necessary	Necessary

Adapted from *Isolation Techniques for Use in Hospitals*. Washington, D.C.: U.S. Government Printing Office, 1970.
*Changed between removal of soiled dressing and application of new dressing.
†Need not be sterile, unless advisable to prevent cross infection of extensive burns or extensive wounds.

necessary. Urine for bacteriological culturing can be collected adequately by cleansing the genitalia prior to the voiding of urine to be sampled. When catheterization is done, it should be for clinical reasons and should always be performed with sterile equipment and with aseptic techniques. The lubricant used must be sterile.

Indwelling urethral catheters should be used only when therapeutically indicated, and the catheter should remain in place only so long as necessary. This procedure should never be done solely for the convenience of doctors and nurses.

A particularly serious complication of catheterization of the urinary tract is the development of septic shock. Fortunately this is not a common complication, but when it occurs prompt antimicrobial and supportive care is essential if death is to be prevented.

General guidelines are as follows:
- Urinary catheterization should be performed only when a physician determines that there is a specific and adequate medical indication.
- Urinary catheterization should be viewed as a minor surgical procedure and aseptic precautions observed.
- Urinary catheterization should be performed only by a physician or by specially trained personnel.
- When an indwelling catheter is used, it should be connected immediately to a sterile closed drainage system.

When a urinary catheterization is performed, the following precautions should be observed:
- The perineum should be adequately exposed and well lighted.
- After the operator has carefully scrubbed his hands, the meatus should be prepared aseptically. This can be done by gently but thoroughly scrubbing the meatus and the immediate surrounding tissues with three successive separate cotton or rayon balls or gauze sponges, soaked in liquid soap or an appropriate disinfectant. This should be followed by a thorough rinse with sterile water.
- After the preparation of the meatus, the operator should don sterile gloves or use a sterile clamp for handling the catheter. Sterile drapes should be used.
- The smallest size sterile catheter that can provide *adequate urinary drainage* (not larger than French no. 18) should be used.
- The catheter should be lubricated with a sterile lubricant, and it is recommended that lubricant also be instilled directly into the urethra. Some physicians may prefer that the sterile lubricant contain an anesthetic.

- If the catheter should touch anything except the sterile gloves, clamp, drapes, or meatus, it must be discarded.
- The catheter must be inserted slowly and carefully to minimize trauma. A traumatic catheterization is likely to result in infection.

The following special considerations are involved in the use of indwelling catheters:

- Several types of catheters are available. The choice should be made by the physician.
- When indwelling catheters are used, the outlet should be connected immediately and aseptically to a sterile closed drainage system. This system should remain intact until the catheter is removed.
- Catheters should not be irrigated unless irrigation is specifically ordered by a physician.
- The three-way catheter permits continuous bladder rinsing with an antimicrobial solution. In select patients this method has been shown to reduce the risk of infection.
- Catheters should not be clamped.
- Drainage bags should be hung from the bed and never inverted or elevated to bladder level.
- Following catheterization the meatal region should be kept clean. Several studies have suggested that daily or more frequent application of an antimicrobial cream to the meatus-catheter junction provides some additional protection against infection.
- Urine specimens can be obtained from the connecting tubing by using a sterile needle and syringe. The area of puncture should be disinfected with iodine or alcohol.
- When it is necessary to change the catheter and drainage system, the new unit should be substituted under the same strict aseptic conditions. Under most circumstances, the interval between changes should not exceed one week.

Observance of these rules of procedure in the performance of catheterizations can be expected to reduce the occurrence of urinary tract infection, and thereby also to reduce the more serious and often fatal bacteremias that result from urinary infections.

Venous catheters

Prolonged intravenous therapy has been greatly facilitated by the availability of small-diameter, flexible plastic catheters. These can be threaded into a peripheral vein to provide a simple means for giving intravenous fluids and medication. Unfortunately, keeping these catheters in place for more than two days often results in septic thrombophlebitis, frequently with dire consequences. In many hospitals, such catheters have been responsible for a significant number of fatal cases of staphylococcal sepsis. Infection by other organisms, such as pseudomonas, streptococci, and candida, has developed similarly. Proper management of these catheters is essential.

Adherence to the following guidelines should minimize the risk of infection whenever intravenous catheters are used. These guidelines apply with equal validity to catheters inserted through a needle and to surgical cutdowns regardless of the site of insertion or the size of the vein being catheterized.

- The skin site should be carefully prepared by scrubbing with a hexachlorophene-containing soap, an iodophor, or tincture of iodine, followed by a 70 per cent alcohol skin prep.
- The site of insertion should be draped as for any surgical procedure.
- The physician who is to insert the catheter should scrub his hands and then don gloves, a gown, and a mask.
- The needle or catheter should be anchored to the site to prevent slippage, mechanical irritation, or introduction of microorganisms.
- Scrupulous aseptic technique should be used when assembling the system or changing fluids.
- Topical neomycin-bacitracin-polymyxin B ointment may be applied to the catheter-skin junction. The site should be covered with an occlusive dry sterile dressing.
- The date of insertion of the catheter should be recorded in a prominent location on the chart.
- The dressing should be removed and the site inspected at least once daily for evidence of local infection or phlebitis. If such is found, the catheter must be removed and, if necessary, a new catheter inserted at a different site. If there is no evidence of local infection or phlebitis, the antibiotic ointment and a fresh dressing should be reapplied.
- The administration set should be changed every 24 hours.
- If the need for intravenous fluid therapy exists for longer than 48 hours, the entire system should be changed and a new needle or catheter inserted at a different site every 48 hours. If a decision is made to leave an intravenous catheter in place for longer than 48 hours, the physician should be fully cognizant of the additional risks of infection being incurred and should justify his decision by a note on the chart. Mere convenience for personnel is not a sufficient reason to incur such risks. The frequency of sepsis resulting from intravenous

fluid therapy is directly related to the length of time a catheter is left in place.

Total parenteral nutrition

Total parenteral nutrition (TPN), or hyperalimentation, is a therapeutic procedure whereby the total body nutritional and fluid requirements are supplied intravenously. This method of feeding is required for patients whose gastrointestinal tracts are nonfunctional as a result of disease or surgical procedures. This technique may also be required if a patient is simply too weak to eat or too emotionally disturbed to take food.

Total parenteral nutrition implies much more than the administration of solutions of sodium chloride, dextrose, bicarbonate, and other electrolytes. The solutions used contain many chemicals and colloids, such as amino acids, carbohydrates, and electrolytes, and thus are usually extremely hypertonic. If the solutions required were introduced into the peripheral veins, thrombophlebitis would result promptly. Therefore, these solutions are administered directly through a flexible catheter into a large deep vein, such as the superior vena cava or the subclavian vein.

Many authors have reported a very high incidence of septicemia during the administration of total parenteral nutrition. Both bacterial and fungal infections have occurred; the latter have been most troublesome and many have been fatal.

Possible sources of these infections are:

- Contamination of the blood stream upon the introduction of the catheter as a result of (a) inadequate surgical asepsis at the time of insertion, (b) a nonsterile catheter, (c) failure to change the infusion sets at 24-hour intervals, or (d) poor technique at the time the set is changed.
- Contamination of the nutritional fluids during preparation and use.
- Leaving the catheter in place for prolonged periods.

To aid in the prevention of infection during total parenteral nutrition, the following practices are helpful:

- The nutrient fluids should be prepared by qualified personnel under aseptic conditions. Commercially prepared nutrition fluids are generally not available except for the ingredients in concentrated form. The ingredients must be mixed and dissolved in sterile pyrogen-free parenteral solutions. Mixing should be done in a unidirectional filtered airflow hood, and the fluid infusion should be completed within 24 hours of preparation.

- Insertion of the catheter should be a surgical procedure. The area of insertion should be thoroughly and vigorously scrubbed. An effective method of skin antisepsis is the use of 1 or 2 per cent tincture of iodine, which is allowed to dry and then removed completely with 70 per cent alcohol. The physician inserting the catheter should be masked, scrubbed, gowned, and gloved. The catheter should be secured in order to avoid motion within the vein during use.

The catheter insertion site should be inspected daily and an appropriate antimicrobial ointment applied. A fresh sterile occlusive dressing is required daily. As long as no signs of local inflammation are noted and no evidence of systemic illness or fever appears, the infusion may be continued without changing the catheter insertion site. If signs of inflammation appear, the catheter must be removed, and the tip and any exudate cultured for bacteria or fungi, and a new sterile catheter inserted at a different site.

Although the likelihood of both local inflammation and septicemia increase with the amount of time the catheter remains in place, the majority may remain for several days without difficulty. The duration of therapy anticipated must be considered in terms of the need for changing the sites, as appropriate sites are not unlimited.

Total parenteral nutrition is a valuable and useful therapeutic tool, despite the problem of serious infection; prevention of such infection requires adherence to predetermined protocol by highly trained personnel.

BIBLIOGRAPHY

INFECTED PERSONNEL AND CARRIERS

Baker, C. J., and Barrett, F. F. Transmission of group B streptococci among parturient women and their neonates. *J. Pediat.* 83:919, Dec. 1973.

Baker, C. J., and others. Suppurative meningitis due to streptococci of Lancefield group B: a study of 33 infants. *J. Pediat.* 82:724, Apr. 1973.

Byrne, E. B. Viral hepatitis: an occupational hazard of medical personnel—experience of the Yale-New Haven Hospital, 1952 to 1965. *J. Amer. Med. Assn.* 195:362, Jan. 31, 1966.

Eickhoff, T. C. Group B streptococci in human infections. In: Wannamaker, L. W., and Matsen, J. M., editors. *Streptococci and Streptococcal Diseases.* New York City: Academic Press, 1972, p. 533.

Eickhoff, T. C., and others. The issue of prophylaxis in neonatal group B streptococcal infections. *J. Pediat.* 83:1097, Dec. 1973.

Hunter, D. T., Jr., and Baker, C. E. Control of staphylococcal carriers in three hospitals. *Pub. Health Rep.* 82:329, Apr. 1967.

McCracken, G. H., Jr. Group B streptococci: The new challenge in neonatal infections. *J. Pediat.* 82:703, Apr. 1973.

Roberts, R. B. *Infections and Sterilization Problems.* Boston: Little, Brown Co., 1972.

HAZARDOUS AREAS

American Academy of Pediatrics. *Care of Children in Hospitals.* 2nd ed. Evanston, Ill.: AAP, 1971.

_____. *Standards and Recommendations for Hospital Care of Newborn Infants.* 5th ed. Evanston, Ill.: AAP, 1971.

American Association of Blood Banks. *Standards for Blood Banks and Transfusion Services.* 5th ed. Chicago: AABB, 1970.

American Hospital Association. *Procedures and Layout for the Infant Formula Room.* Chicago: AHA, 1965.

Creutzfeldt, W., and others. Transmission of hepatitis over 10 years by a blood donor with posthepatic cirrhosis. *German Med. Monthly.* 8:30, Jan. 1963.

Findlay, C. W., Jr. Sepsis in the surgical intensive care unit. *Med. Clin. N. Amer.* 55:1331, Sept. 1971.

Krugman, S., and others. Infectious hepatitis. *J. Amer. Med. Assn.* 200:365, May 1, 1967.

Mosley, J. W. Prevention of post-transfusional viral hepatitis. *Hospitals, J.A.H.A.* 39:94, July 16, 1965.

National Academy of Sciences—National Research Council. *General Principles of Blood Transfusion.* Washington, D.C.: NAS, 1963.

_____. *The Incidence, Mortality, and Prevention of Post-Transfusion Hepatitis.* A review prepared by the Committee on Plasma and Plasma Substitutes of the Division of Medical Sciences, National Research Council. Washington, D.C.: NAS, June 1965.

Segal, S., and others. *Transport of High Risk Newborn Infants.* Vancouver, B.C.: Canadian Paediatric Society, 1972.

HAZARDOUS PROCEDURES

Bassett, D. C. J., and others. Neonatal infections with *pseudomonas aeruginosa* associated with contaminated resuscitation equipment. *Lancet.* (1):781, Apr. 10, 1965.

Bentley, D. W., and Lepper, M. H. Septicemia related to indwelling venous catheters. *J. Amer. Med. Assn.* 206:1749, Nov. 18, 1968.

Edmondson, E. B. Pseudomonas in gas therapy and aerosol equipment. *Lancet.* (1):660, Mar. 1966.

Elek, S. D., and Conen, P. E. The virulence of *staphylococcus pyogenes* for man. A study of the problem of wound infection. *Brit. J. Exp. Path.* 38:573, Dec. 1957.

Gibbons, C. P. Care of anesthesia equipment. *Hosp. Top.* 42:109, Sept. 1964.

Herman, L., and Himmelsbach, C. K. Detection and control of hospital sources of flavobacteria. *Hospitals, J.A.H.A.* 39:72, June 16, 1965.

Kass, E. H. *Progress in Pyelonephritis.* Philadelphia: F. A. Davis, 1965.

Kunin, C. M., and McCormack, R. C. Prevention of catheter-induced urinary tract infections by sterile, closed drainage. *N. Eng. J. Med.* 274:1155, May 26, 1966.

Martin, C. M., and Bookrajian, E. N. Bacteriuria prevention after indwelling urinary catheterization. A controlled study. *Arch. Int. Med.* 110:703, Nov. 1962.

Meyers, M. S., and others. Controlled trial of nitrofurazone and neomycin-polymyxin as constant bladder rinses for prevention of post-indwelling catheterization bacteriuria. In: Sylvester, J. C., editor. *Antimicrobial Agents and Chemotherapy—1964.* Ann Arbor, Mich.: American Society for Microbiology, 1965.

Pierce, A. K., and Sanford, J. P. Control of microbial contamination of inhalation therapy equipment. In: *Proceedings of the International Conference on Nosocomial Infections.* Chicago: American Hospital Association, 1971, pp. 255-58.

Prevention of Urinary Tract Infection from Catheters. 16-mm, sound, color, 30-min. film. Tuckahoe, N.Y.: Burroughs Wellcome & Co., Inc., 1967.

Reinarz, J. A., and others. The potential role of inhalation therapy equipment in nosocomial pulmonary infection. *J. Clin. Invest.* 44:831, May 1965.

Rittenberg, M. S., and Hench, M. E. Evaluation of activated glutaraldehyde. *Ann. Surg.* 161:127, Jan. 1965.

Ross, P. W. A new disinfectant: activated glutaraldehyde. *J. Clin. Pathol.* (UK) 19:318, July 1966.

Sanford, J. P. Hospital acquired urinary infections. *Ann. Int. Med.* 60:903, May 1964.

Sanford, J. P., and Pierce, A. K. Current infection problems—respiratory. In: *Proceedings of the International Conference on Nosocomial Infections.* Chicago: American Hospital Association, 1971, pp. 77-81.

Snow, J. C., and others. Sterilization of anesthesia equipment with ethylene oxide. *N. Eng. J. Med.* 266:443, Mar. 1, 1962.

Stamey, T. A. *Renovascular Hypertension.* Baltimore: Williams & Wilkins, 1963.

Stratford, B. C., and others. Disinfection of anesthetic apparatus. *Brit. J. Anes.* 36:471, Aug. 1964.

Vanamee, P., and others. *Symposium on Total Parenteral Nutrition.* Chicago: American Medical Association (Food Science Committee), 1972.

Epilog

OBSERVATIONS ON MOTIVATION

> A mighty creature is the germ
> Though smaller than a pachyderm.
> His customary dwelling place
> Is deep within the human race.
> His childish pride he often pleases
> By giving people strange diseases.
>
> *Ogden Nash*

Although hospital programs for the prevention and control of nosocomial infections have improved, they are not as good as they should be nor as effective as they will be if the guidelines proposed in this manual are taken seriously. In the original and revised versions of this handbook, the Committee on Infections Within Hospitals attempted to:
- Identify and describe those factors and conditions that tend to foster contagion and to permit its spread.
- Describe how to organize and operate an effective program for the control and prevention of nosocomial infections.
- Emphasize the legal and professional obligations of every hospital to maintain an effective infection control program.
- Charge the full-time and attending clinical staffs of hospitals with an equal share of responsibility for the prevention and control of nosocomial infections.

- Stress the importance of teaching all hospital personnel *what* they need to know about microbial contamination and the spread of infection in their respective areas of work, and *how* to perform their tasks in a fashion that will eliminate or substantially reduce these dangers.

The committee recognized that the success of such an infection control program depends on the proper participation of all hospital personnel. Not only must these personnel have a sufficiently clear grasp of the physical and biological factors essential to good control measures in their work, but also they must translate this knowledge into action. This takes both skill and motivation. Skill can be taught, but the desire and the will to do the right thing—especially when it requires additional effort—must come from within. The factors that motivate good human behavior are both complex and individual; those factors that have to do with pride in playing a role in the healing arts, with bettering, compassion, and caring, should be cultivated and reinforced in hospital personnel.

But in addition to building on those factors that tend to influence good behavior, it is necessary to counteract those that act conversely. One negative motivational problem relates to the fact that the satisfaction a person derives from the proper performance of measures for prevention and control of infection can never equal or compete with the satisfaction associated with curing the illness of a sick person. Nevertheless, it should be kept in mind that many of the dramatic aspects of modern curative medicine could not even be attempted with safety if it were not for the effectiveness of modern measures for the prevention and control of nosocomial infections. Other influences that tend to operate negatively on motivation include the facts that:

- Neither the presence of microbes nor evidence of breaks in aseptic techniques is visible to the naked eye. Thus, out of sight too often means, literally, out of mind. Training programs should emphasize the importance of relying on the mind's eye whenever the naked eye doesn't suffice.
- The latent period between a break in technique and the appearance of a nosocomial infection is too great to convince the culprit that a direct cause-and-effect relationship exists. Efforts should be made to inculcate an appreciation that the usual cause of nosocomial infection is a break in aseptic technique, somewhere along the line. It should also be pointed out, however, that not all breaks in aseptic technique result in infection, but that this fortuitous circumstance can and often does lead to a false sense of security and to a disbelief in the essentiality of medical asepsis.

Such negative influences may operate to undermine the practice of asepsis, especially in the presence of glaring examples of disregard by nonconformist leaders. Success in the prevention and control of nosocomial infections depends on hospital workers' unshakable belief that no microbe is capable of penetrating our defenses if we keep them adequate. The name of the game is prevention.

Appendix A

STATEMENT ON CARE OF PATIENTS WITH PULMONARY TUBERCULOSIS IN GENERAL HOSPITALS

INTRODUCTION

Medical progress during the past two decades has had a major impact on the patterns of health care delivery to patients with tuberculosis. Important factors that have contributed to these changes are the highly effective antituberculosis chemotherapeutic agents presently available and a better understanding of the epidemiology of that disease, particularly with reference to its infectiousness. As a result, it has become both medically and economically unreasonable to maintain large numbers of tuberculosis hospitals. Rather, it has become increasingly apparent that the general hospital is the logical place to admit tuberculosis patients who need hospitalization, whether for tuberculosis or some other concurrent or complicating illness. To ensure that patients with tuberculosis are given optimal care, only those hospitals willing to provide the necessary services should consider assuming this responsibility (ref. 1).

The following procedures and policies are offered as a guide to general hospitals to facilitate the assumption of responsibility for care of patients with tuberculosis.

Approved by American Hospital Association and National Tuberculosis and Respiratory Disease Association, Nov. 17-19, 1971.

ROLE OF THE INFECTION CONTROL COMMITTEE

Close supervision by the infection control committee will be necessary to ensure that tuberculosis patients receive a quality of care equivalent to that given patients with other diseases and to ensure that the presence in the hospital of patients with tuberculosis does not present a risk to other patients or staff.

The committee should give particular attention to the following:

1. Provision of an inservice educational program for all professional and allied health personnel to provide a better understanding of the management of patients with tuberculosis and to provide factual knowledge of the epidemiology and methods of transmission of tuberculosis. Information and assistance in the development of programs may be obtained by contacting the local Tuberculosis and Respiratory Disease Association.*
2. Provision of necessary inhospital services, with particular attention to nursing, laboratory, radiology, and social services.
3. Anticipation of questions from the community regarding the infectiousness of tuberculosis and the measures being taken to protect other patients, visitors, and hospital staff from acquiring tuberculosis.

INHOSPITAL SERVICES

Because of advances in diagnosis and treatment, it is no longer necessary to admit all tuberculosis patients to hospitals. The focus of care of the tuberculosis patient is now the outpatient facility, clinic, health center, or physician's office, where the patient should receive most, and sometimes all, of his treatment. Advances in diagnostic techniques make hospitalization solely for diagnostic purposes unnecessary in most instances. Patients who may still require hospitalization include those who are symptomatically ill, those with other major diseases, those who present complex diagnostic problems, those who present difficult problems in the selection and maintenance of chemotherapy programs, and those who are considered infectious for others. Extended hospitalization, however, is rarely required. The decision as to which patients should be hospitalized will vary somewhat among individual physicians (ref. 2).

Before a general hospital assumes responsibility for tuberculosis patients, the infection control committee must make sure that the necessary inpatient and outpatient services are available. These services include:

---

*Now the American Lung Association.

1. The availability of beds to which patients with tuberculosis will be admitted.
2. The availability of a physician with expertise in the management of tuberculosis and who is well informed about the community facilities and services available.
3. Adequate consultative services, either within or outside the hospital.
4. The availability of laboratory services competent in the biochemical and bacteriologic techniques needed to diagnose and evaluate tuberculosis.
5. The availability of necessary radiologic services.
6. An interested, understanding, and informed nursing staff.
7. The availability of necessary outpatient services and follow-up.

The most important ingredient is an attitude—a willingness and a desire on the part of all members of the hospital staff to provide high-quality care to all its patients.

SPECIFIC MEASURES NECESSARY IN THE HOSPITAL CARE OF TUBERCULOSIS PATIENTS DURING COMMUNICABILITY

Three factors should be considered in determining the communicability of tuberculosis: pulmonary cavitation, cough and sputum production, and the presence of acid-fast bacilli on a direct smear of the sputum concentrate. The communicability of tuberculosis has been shown to be primarily a result of airborne transmission, usually by means of droplet nuclei from unprotected coughing and sneezing of patients with open (positive on direct smear) pulmonary tuberculosis (ref. 3). For this reason, respiratory isolation is the appropriate form of isolation during the period of communicability, and procedures used should conform to those specified for respiratory isolation (ref. 4). If the proper precautions against airborne spread are maintained by patients in isolation, visitors need not be subject to restrictions or special precautions.

The first and most important measure against the spread of infection is education of the *patient* on how to avoid contaminating his immediate atmospheric environment. He should be taught to be scrupulous in covering his mouth with disposable paper tissues when coughing, raising sputum, or sneezing. Sputum ordinarily should be spit into paper tissues. All tissues should be placed in paper bags to be incinerated or disposed of in the same way as other contaminated material.

If the infectious patient is unable or unwilling to cover his mouth during coughing, expectoration, or sneezing, he should wear a mask covering both nose and mouth. The high-efficiency disposable masks are more effective than the standard cotton gauze masks in preventing airborne and droplet spread.

Patients with tuberculosis must be separated from other patients, either in private rooms or in larger rooms restricted to those with tuberculosis. Masks and gowns are not needed under usual circumstances for patients themselves, for hospital personnel, or for visitors.

Good ventilation without recirculation of air is essential for rooms or wards used for tuberculosis patients. If ventilation of rooms in which there are patients with sputum-positive pulmonary tuberculosis permits air to flow into the corridor or adjacent rooms, window exhaust fans should be installed so that room air will be discharged directly to the outside. Care should be taken that such exhausted air does not reenter the hospital through nearby open windows or air intakes.

Ultraviolet light is not a requirement in areas where tuberculosis patients are under treatment. Properly installed and maintained, however, ultraviolet lights will help to reduce numbers of airborne mycobacteria that circulate within inches of these lights. The use of ultraviolet light must not be allowed to become a substitute for precautionary measures such as controlling cough and expectoration by the patient. At the same time, it should be realized that ultraviolet lights, installed for maximum effect on airborne microorganisms, will not kill mycobacteria in dried particles of mucus on such surfaces as floors, tables, or bed frames.

Fomites do not constitute a significant hazard; therefore *special* laundering, dishwashing, or cleaning procedures are not necessary. Items such as books, magazines, and newspapers can be handled in the ordinary way and need not be restricted from subsequent use by other patients.

Proper housekeeping procedures should be carried out at least daily, as they are for all hospital rooms. A detergent-germicide with good tuberculocidal activity such as a chlorophenol (2 per cent) or an iodophore (450-ppm. strength) is suggested.

Terminal cleaning procedures after discharge of a patient with tuberculosis need be no different from those carried out in any other room. In the case of patients for whom respiratory isolation was required, terminal cleaning procedures should conform to those recommended for that category of isolation (ref. 4).

The elaborate prolonged isolation procedures recommended in the past are unnecessary in the present era of chemotherapy. The period of communicability of tuberculosis is sharply reduced within a relatively short period of time after effective treatment has begun. Within two to three weeks after the patient has been started on effective chemotherapy, the infectivity of his respiratory secretions will usually have diminished enough for him to be removed from isolation. There are currently no quantitative criteria to document this, but a substantial reduction in the number of bacilli in the sputum, as observed in a direct smear of the sputum concentrate, is to be expected. There should by then have been a clinical response to therapy, with a decrease in cough, sputum production, and fever. These clinical signs can be used as a guide for termination of isolation precautions (ref. 5).

Tuberculosis patients need not be segregated as a public health measure except during the period of communicability. Grouping of patients in a special room or area is recommended primarily to facilitate their instruction and orientation, supervision of the taking of medication, and to ensure that they will come under the observation and care of physicians with particular expertise in the treatment of tuberculosis. Particular care must be exercised, however, to ensure that patients are not denied adequate diagnostic and therapeutic services for nontuberculosis conditions as a result of segregation in a special tuberculosis unit.

The greatest risk to contacts of patients having open pulmonary tuberculosis occurs during the period before the disease has been recognized.

TUBERCULOSIS SURVEILLANCE OF HOSPITAL STAFF

A tuberculosis control program is necessary as part of employee health services regardless of whether or not tuberculosis patients are knowingly admitted. Inevitably, some persons with active tuberculosis will be admitted for treatment of other diseases without immediate recognition of the presence of tuberculosis. Such unrecognized cases constitute the greatest hazard of tuberculosis infection for hospital personnel.

The preemployment physical examination should include a standard chest x-ray and a tuberculin skin test using 5 T.U. PPD. Tuberculin-negative employees should have repeat skin tests at least annually, and more often if in intimate or prolonged contact with infectious patients. Tuberculin-positive employees should have repeat chest films at least annually. *If an employee's tuberculin reaction converts from negative to positive, a medical evaluation is indicated. It is strongly recommended that the employee be given isoniazid for a one-year period* (ref. 6).

REPORTING AND POSTHOSPITAL CARE

Ultimate responsibility for medical follow-up rests with the patient's physician or with an appropriate public or private clinic. The reporting of confirmed cases is required by law because public health authorities are responsible for tuberculosis control. In many places, reporting of suspect cases is also required by law or regulation. Such reporting will initiate the cooperation of the health department in the screening and surveillance of contacts and in an epidemiological investigation to determine the source of the patient's infection.

Prior to discharge, a plan should be formulated in concert with the health department for the patient's subsequent outpatient care. All necessary measures should be taken to ensure that the patient will continue to take medication on an outpatient basis. Such planning may require specific discussion with the public health authorities, the Visiting Nurse Association, and others. In each hospital, a procedure should be established to ensure that a copy of the patient's discharge clinical summary is supplied to the physician or clinic responsible for his follow-up care and to the appropriate public health jurisdiction.

SUMMARY

Greater recognition of the responsibility to treat patients with tuberculosis in general hospitals is highly desirable, but such recognition carries with it specific obligations to the patient with tuberculosis to other patients, to hospital personnel, and to the community at large. With this statement as a guideline, the infection control committee should assume major responsibility for this transition to the benefit of patients with tuberculosis, to the hospital, and to the community at large.

BIBLIOGRAPHY

1. National Tuberculosis and Respiratory Disease Association. Guidelines for the general hospital in the admission and care of tuberculosis patients. *Amer. Rev. Resp. Dis.* 99:631, Apr. 1969.
2. Mitchell, R. S., and others. Standards for tuberculosis treatment in the 1970s. *Amer. Rev. Resp. Dis.* 102:992, Dec. 1970.
3. Olsen A. M., and others. Infectiousness of tuberculosis in general hospitals. *Amer. Rev. Resp. Dis.* 96:836, Oct. 1967
4. U.S. National Communicable Disease Center. *Isolation Techniques for Use in Hospitals* (Public Health Service Publication No. 2054). Washington, D.C.: U.S. Government Printing Office, 1970.
5. Wolinsky, E., and others. Bacteriologic standards for the discharge of patients. *Amer. Rev. Resp. Dis.* 102:470, Sept. 1970.
6. American Hospital Association. *Infection Control in the Hospital.* Chicago: AHA, 1970.
7. American Thoracic Society, National Tuberculosis and Respiratory Disease Association, and the U.S. Public Health Service. Preventive treatment of tuberculosis. *Amer. Rev. Resp. Dis.* 104:460, Sept. 1971.
8. American Thoracic Society. Personnel tuberculosis control program in medical institutions. *Amer. Rev. Resp. Dis.* 104:463, Sept. 1971.

Appendix B

STATEMENT ON MICROBIOLOGIC SAMPLING IN THE HOSPITAL

The focal point of hospital infection control must necessarily be the patient: both the patient who already has an infection and the patient who does not have an infection but is at risk of acquiring one. In either instance, measures must be directed toward preventing spread of infection from any source to noninfected personnel or patients. It is from this point of view that microbiologic sampling must be considered and its value judged.

Routine environmental microbiologic sampling programs are those programs conducted on a regularly scheduled basis. They include sampling of air, surfaces, linens, fomites, and so forth in patient care areas, surgical suites, and nurseries irrespective of specific nosocomial infection problems. It is obvious that infection control authorities wish to ensure that housekeeping practices within the hospital will maintain a clean and safe environment for patients. Procedures used by the nursing, housekeeping, laundry, dietary, and maintenance departments need to be examined in those terms by the infection committee. Certain areas, such as surgical suites, nurseries, intensive care, and dialysis units, and certain procedures known to be associated with increased risk of infection require special

---

Approved by American Hospital Association, Nov. 14-18, 1973.

attention. Examples of such procedures are urinary tract and intravenous catheterization, tracheostomies, and inhalation therapy.

The Committee on Infections Within Hospitals finds no evidence that *routine* environmental sampling is necessary to maintain good practices in the hospital, nor is there evidence that this type of *routine* sampling has contributed significantly to the prevention of nosocomial infection. The occurrence or prevalence of nosocomial infection has not been related to levels of microbial contamination of air, surfaces, and fomites, and meaningful standards for permissible levels of such contamination do not exist.

The Committee on Infections Within Hospitals is of the opinion that *routine* microbiologic sampling of the hospital environment, done with no specific epidemiologic goal in mind, is unnecessary and economically unjustifiable. Unfortunately, in many hospitals, environmental sampling programs appear to have taken the place of infection surveillance programs. As a result, in some hospitals the infection committee and hospital administration have acquired much uninterpretable and often irrelevant data about the levels of microbial contamination on floors, walls, and linens and in the air, but little or no knowledge of the frequency of occurrence of hospital-acquired infection.

Microbiologic sampling of the hospital environment must, therefore, always be a means to an end and never an end in itself. What role should microbiologic sampling play in the total picture of hospital infection control?

The most useful role of microbiologic sampling lies in the investigation of specific problems within the hospital, and here it should be considered a necessary adjunct to the infection control program. For example, if a cluster of similar cases or a frank epidemic occurs in which epidemiologic evidence leads the infection committee to suspect particular articles, such as nebulizer bottles, solutions, endotracheal tubes, antiseptics, or the like, as the source of infection, microbiologic sampling should be carried out under the direction of the hospital epidemiologist. The hospital epidemiologist should indicate the numbers, types, and sources of samples to be taken as well as the specific microorganisms being sought based on the epidemiologic evidence.

Should outbreaks of staphylococcal, streptococcal, or salmonella infection occur, microbiologic sampling of personnel would similarly be an appropriate procedure to employ. Epidemiologic evidence has sometimes implicated personnel in the nosocomial spread of other gram-negative bacilli, such as *Klebsiella, Proteus,* or *Pseudomonas*. Microbiologic sampling of personnel is an appropriate investigative tool in such a situation. All microbiologic screening of personnel should be directed and guided by the hospital epidemiologist, in the light of total epidemiologic information. Such application of microbiologic sampling techniques has proved highly useful in the investigation of a case or cluster of cases in which there is a reasonable possibility, on the basis of epidemiologic evidence, of an identifiable exogenous source.

The Committee on Infections Within Hospitals recognizes the necessity for carrying out a certain number of routine sampling procedures as quality control checks of sterilization procedures. Such testing of the effectiveness of procedures would include the measurement of microbial content of hospital-prepared infant formulas and standardized tests for sterility, plus batch sampling when indicated. Several investigators have emphasized the importance of occasional spot-checking of certain patient care equipment known to be associated with a high risk of hospital-acquired infection. Sampling of nebulizer reservoirs of inhalation therapy equipment is a commonly cited example. Such sampling procedures may be particularly useful if cleaning methods as usage procedures are changed. The risk of hospital-associated infection occurring from such equipment or from contaminated antiseptics is more effectively controlled by enforcing rigid adherence to tested protocols covering preparation, disinfection or preferably sterilization, length of use, and maintenance, rather than by *routine* sampling procedures.

Environmental sampling programs are sometimes said to be useful in personnel education and training. Although this may be true, it is the opinion of the committee that the educational value of such programs is quickly lost if the sampling programs are allowed to become *routine,* perfunctory duties carried out with no relation to specific nosocomial infection problems.

The epidemiology of many nosocomial infections is still poorly understood, and there are many valid research applications of environmental sampling techniques. Whether there are reservoirs within the hospital of organisms such as *Candida, Aspergillus, Nocardia,* and other emerging pathogens is not yet clear. The spread of viruses within hospitals has been little studied. The intrahospital reservoirs of multidrug-resistant strains of *Klebsiella, Serratia,* and other organisms commonly acquired by patients during hospitalization are not completely understood. These are but a few epidemiologic problems, study of which often necessarily includes microbiologic sampling procedures.

In summary, microbiologic sampling procedures, if carried out when indicated in the investigation of specific epidemiologic problems, can be extremely helpful in the control of nosocomial infections. Similarly, quality control of disinfection or sterilization procedures is justified on a planned basis, particularly when new methods are introduced. Much research remains to be done in order to define possible reservoirs within the hospital of many organisms associated with nosocomial infection. *Routine* microbiologic sampling of the hospital environment, however, not only has provided data that are impossible to interpret but also has contributed little to hospital infection control.

The Committee on Infections Within Hospitals concludes that *routine* environmental sampling is unnecessary and wasteful.

Appendix C

GUIDELINES ON TUBERCULOSIS CONTROL PROGRAMS FOR HOSPITAL EMPLOYEES

INTRODUCTION

Recent statements from the American Lung Association (formerly the National Tuberculosis and Respiratory Disease Association), the American College of Chest Physicians, and the American Hospital Association have dealt with the increasingly greater role that general hospitals play in the primary care of patients with tuberculosis (ref. 1-3). The need for a tuberculosis control program as a part of personnel health services has been emphasized in these statements.

The responsibility for ensuring that an effective tuberculosis control program is carried out is properly a function of the hospital infection control committee. In the development of such a program, it is important that the hospital administration, the infection control committee, and the physicians charged with the care of hospital personnel be aware of the options available in protecting against tuberculosis and decide which approach best suits the immediate needs in a given locale. This statement provides background information and guidelines to establish such a program.

Approved by American Hospital Association General Council, Oct. 25, 1974.

RISK AMONG HOSPITAL PERSONNEL

Unrecognized cases constitute the greatest hazard of tuberculosis infection for hospital personnel and for patients. Therefore surveillance of hospital staff members for tuberculosis is necessary whether or not patients with tuberculosis are knowingly admitted to the hospital.

It is inevitable that some persons with active tuberculosis are admitted for treatment of other illnesses without immediate recognition of the presence of tuberculosis. This risk can be reduced but not totally eliminated if chest x-rays are obtained routinely upon admission. In addition, in patients with certain viral infections, such as measles, or in patients receiving corticosteroid or other immunosuppressive therapy, a positive tuberculin test may be rendered negative and thus make the presence of tuberculosis more difficult to recognize. In other instances tuberculosis may be reactivated as a result of immunosuppressive diseases or therapy and thus may constitute a hazard to hospital personnel.

The number of persons with unrecognized cases of tuberculosis admitted to hospitals will be greatest in communities or areas in which there is a relatively high endemic incidence of tuberculosis. Employees of hospitals serving urban areas, particularly those with large skid row or ghetto populations, in which the endemic incidence of tuberculosis is higher than in other sectors of the population, can expect to encounter tuberculosis frequently among fellow employees as well as among their patients. It is therefore particularly important for the hospital serving such an area to develop and maintain an effective program of tuberculosis surveillance of its personnel.

Personnel involved in providing direct patient care are subject to the greatest risk of acquiring tuberculosis. They include physicians, nurses, practical nurses, aides, and other patient care personnel whose activities bring them into frequent, close contact with patients who have tuberculosis, diagnosed and undiagnosed.

The risk to other groups of hospital personnel decreases as the frequency of their patient contacts decreases. Laboratory personnel processing specimens such as sputum from patients known to have or suspected of having tuberculosis are not subject to increased risk if standard laboratory precautions are observed. Just as the greatest hazard to patient care personnel is the patient with unsuspected tuberculosis, the greatest hazard to laboratory personnel is the casual handling of specimens from such a patient.

In contrast to the circumstances three or four decades ago, when most hospital personnel were tuberculin positive, hospital personnel in the 1970s are 65 per cent to 90 per cent tuberculin negative. A negative tuberculin test strongly suggests, but does not prove, that the individual has never acquired a tuberculous infection. A positive tuberculin test indicates that the person has a delayed type of hypersensitivity to the tubercle bacillus or its products and that at some time in the past he had a tuberculosis infection. Individuals who are tuberculin negative are susceptible to exogenous infection, whereas those who are tuberculin positive are resistant to exogenous infection but are particularly subject to reactivation of their original tuberculous infection. Therefore, among hospital personnel, the tuberculin-negative group runs the risk of acquiring primary tuberculosis from someone else and the tuberculin-positive group runs the risk of developing "reactivation" tuberculosis (ref. 4, 5).

APPROACHES TO SURVEILLANCE AND CONTROL

Tuberculin Skin Testing and Isoniazid Prophylaxis

Tuberculin skin testing and isoniazid prophylaxis constitute the most widely recommended approach to tuberculosis control in American hospitals.

Initial examination

The preemployment physical examination should include a standard chest x-ray and tuberculin skin test (Mantoux test) using 5 TU tuberculin purified protein derivative (PPD, Tween stabilized). A positive test is defined as induration of 10 millimeters or more at 48 hours. The multiple-puncture technique (Tine test) may also be used, but the intradermal tuberculin test is preferred, because of its superior standardization.

False negative reactions to PPD may occur. The use of PPD stabilized with Tween-80 and the administration of the solution immediately after it is drawn into glass or plastic syringes minimize the frequency of false negative reactions (ref. 6).

Follow-up of tuberculin-negative employees

Tuberculin-negative employees should have skin tests at least annually, but every six months if in intimate or prolonged contact with known infectious patients. Surveillance of tuberculin-negative personnel with exposure to known infectious tuberculosis patients should consist of tuberculin skin testing at six-month intervals. On occasion, primary prophylactic isoniazid therapy may be indicated for a tuberculin-negative employee with unusually extensive exposure to a tuberculosis patient who is excreting large numbers of bacilli. These employees should be skin tested at the outset. If they are still negative after three months of isoniazid therapy, the isoniazid therapy may be discontinued.

Management of tuberculin converters

If an employee's tuberculin reaction, previously negative, is found on follow-up testing to have become positive, a diagnosis of tuberculous infection should be made and a full medical evaluation carried out. If active clinical tuberculosis is found, the employee should be treated with at least two drugs for two years, in accordance with current practice. If there is no evidence of tuberculous disease, the employee *should be given preventive isoniazid treatment for one year* (ref. 7).

Follow-up of employees initially tuberculin positive

An employee found to be tuberculin positive on initial examination should have a chest x-ray annually, or more often if clinically indicated. Preventive treatment with isoniazid is not recommended for a person who is tuberculin positive on initial examination, except under certain clinical circumstances known to carry an increased risk of reactivation of latent tuberculosis. These circumstances include the presence of: abnormal chest x-rays, consistent with inactive tuberculosis; diabetes mellitus; corticosteroid or other immunosuppressive therapy; gastrectomy; or underlying reticuloendothelial disease, such as Hodgkin's disease.

The decision to give preventive isoniazid treatment to a tuberculin-positive employee must be made on an individual basis by the responsible physician. Isoniazid treatment is not wholly without risk, and recently attention has been called to its potential hepatotoxicity (ref. 8-10). Should latent tuberculous infection be reactivated, however, the risk of tuberculosis extends beyond the employee to the patients. Accordingly, isoniazid treatment is fully justified for the groups described above. In contrast, for the otherwise healthy employee whose tuberculin test is positive on initial examination and whose chest x-ray is normal, isoniazid treatment is not recommended.

BCG (Bacille Calmette-Guerin) Vaccine

An alternative approach to control of tuberculosis among hospital employees is the use of Bacille Calmette-Guerin (BCG) vaccine in tuberculin-negative individuals.

The rationale for this approach is that tuberculin-negative individuals run the risk of acquiring primary tuberculous disease, which at times can be rapidly progressive. Protection against that risk is obtained by activating the cellular immune mechanisms of the host to the antigens contained in BCG vaccine. These antigens are closely related, but not identical, to those of virulent *Mycobacterium tuberculosis*. Vaccination with BCG usually changes a person's tuberculin test from negative to positive.

This approach calls for new personnel to have both a standard chest x-ray and a tuberculin skin test using 5 TU PPD as part of their pre-employment physical examination. Tuberculin-negative personnel are then given BCG vaccine and thereafter should have repeat chest x-rays annually, or more often if clinically indicated. The need for follow-up skin testing of personnel who receive BCG vaccine is controversial. This may be carried out six weeks after vaccination, to ascertain whether skin-test conversion has occurred. It is not considered necessary to reimmunize with BCG in order to achieve protection if the skin test remains negative. Repeated annual skin tests, however, are not necessary. The employee should be informed on a card or other suitable immunization record that he has been given BCG vaccine. There is no danger in the administration of BCG vaccine to tuberculin-positive employees, although such use of the vaccine is unnecessary.

BCG vaccine may be used on an optional basis for tuberculin-negative personnel. Personnel made tuberculin positive by BCG should have annual chest x-rays, and unvaccinated tuberculin-negative personnel should have periodic skin tests as outlined under Follow-up of Tuberculin-Negative Employees.

Prior to embarking on a BCG program, each hospital should assess the tuberculosis risk among its personnel. It should be recognized in such assessment that each employee represents, in addition to the hospital risk, that risk incurred from the community in which he resides. A BCG program should be considered only if the tuberculin conversion rate in personnel is found to exceed one per cent annually. It is essential to confirm a specific hospital risk prior to initiating a BCG program.

INFORMATION ON ISONIAZID

Isoniazid is a highly effective bactericidal antituberculosis agent, which is a component of most tuberculosis treatment regimens. Extensive experience has also demonstrated its effectiveness in preventing clinical tuberculosis in infected individuals. Preventive treatment is utilized by most, if not all, local health departments in the United States. A joint statement of the

American Thoracic Society, the American Lung Association, and the Center for Disease Control outlines the rationale and methods for use of isoniazid preventive treatment (ref. 7). Approximately 650,000 individuals are provided preventive treatment in the United States annually.

The U.S. Public Health Service has conducted six prophylaxis trials since 1955, involving almost 70,000 persons (ref. 11). Each trial has matched isoniazid therapy at 5 milligrams per kilogram of body weight against a placebo medication. The six trials have involved children with primary tuberculosis; Alaskan villagers; childhood and adult contacts; mental patients; and individuals with healed, previously untreated tuberculous lesions. In the six trials there have been a cumulative reduction in clinical tuberculosis of 61 per cent during the treatment year (range of 18 per cent to 95 per cent) and a continued cumulative reduction over 14 years of follow-up of approximately 50 per cent.

It is therefore reasonable to expect a 50 per cent to 75 per cent reduction in clinical tuberculosis when high-risk groups of infected individuals, such as hospital personnel who have recently converted from tuberculin negative to positive, are treated with isoniazid for one year.

Isoniazid is well suited for preventive therapy because of the low incidence of side effects associated with its administration. Infrequent problems that may arise are peripheral neuropathy, an increased frequency of seizures in patients with convulsive disorders, a syndrome simulating systemic lupus erythematosis, and hepatitis. The first two problems are related to competitive inhibition of utilization of pyridoxine by neural tissue. This effect can be blocked by the administration of 50 milligrams of pyridoxine per day to patients prone to either disorder, although its prevention in patients with convulsive disorders is less well established. The lupus syndrome is very rare and is usually alleviated by withdrawal of the drug. The incidence of hepatitis remains debatable and is under detailed prospective evaluation at the present time. Serious sequelae, including death, have been encountered very rarely and not at all in many cities treating many thousands of patients with isoniazid. It has yet to be confirmed that minor elevations of liver enzyme values reflect a direct effect of isoniazid or, if they do, whether they represent a harmful effect (ref. 8).

In summary, isoniazid chemoprophylaxis is a safe and effective method for preventing clinical tuberculosis among infected individuals. Combined with an effectively applied tuberculin skin testing program, it is the drug of choice for preventive therapy in a population with a low tuberculous infection and conversion rate.

INFORMATION ON BCG VACCINE

BCG vaccine is widely used as a primary form of tuberculosis control in many countries, particularly those in which the endemic incidence of tuberculosis is high. The use of this product in the United States has been limited and has long been a controversial issue among clinicians, epidemiologists, public health administrators, and others charged with responsibility for the control of tuberculosis.

The U.S. Public Health Service, on the basis of a statement prepared by its consultants, has recommended against the use of BCG vaccine among medical or paramedical personnel (ref. 12). Similarly, the American Thoracic Society has not recommended the use of BCG vaccine among hospital personnel (ref. 13). On the basis of the same evidence, other experts have disputed this view and recommended the use of BCG vaccine among exposed populations such as selected hospital personnel (ref. 14-17).

The safety of BCG vaccine is not questioned. Earlier concerns about hazards have long since been dispelled, and extensive worldwide use of BCG vaccine has adequately documented its safety. However, as with other live attenuated immunogens, its use should be avoided in immunologically incompetent hosts, such as those with lymphoreticular malignancies or individuals being given immunosuppressive therapy, because cases of overt disease due to infection with the attenuated BCG organism in such individuals have been reported.

The effectiveness of BCG vaccine has been established in a number of studies, both in the United States and abroad. Reports by Rosenthal (ref. 18), Aronson (ref. 19), Dickie (ref. 20), Frimodt-Møller (ref. 21), and the Medical Research Council of Great Britain (ref. 22) have confirmed that BCG vaccine provides 60 per cent to 80 per cent protection against pulmonary tuberculosis over a 10-year period as compared to nonvaccinated tuberculin-negative controls. In contrast, however, studies reported by Comstock and Palmer (ref. 23) and Comstock and Webster (ref. 24), carried out in rural areas of Georgia and Alabama, showed a reduction in active tuberculosis of only 14 per cent among BCG vaccinated children. There are thus well-authenticated differences in effectiveness of BCG vaccines in various studies, which may depend in part on the specific BCG vaccines used, the effect of natural immunization by atypical mycobacteria, and the risk of tuberculosis in the population under study.

The arguments against the use of BCG vaccine are based on the following observations: (1) the greatest risk of overt, active tuberculosis resides in the tuberculin-positive population, and this risk would not be diminished by the use of BCG; (2) the risk of hospital personnel being exposed to tuberculosis is steadily declining; and (3) immunization with BCG interferes with the use of the tuberculin test as a case-finding technique. The tuberculin test is helpful in the differential diagnosis of pulmonary abnormalities, including bronchogenic carcinoma and other nontuberculous conditions.

Proponents of the use of BCG vaccine in selected population groups, such as hospital personnel, base their arguments on (1) its known safety and efficacy; (2) the fact that tuberculosis is still a significant endemic problem in many large urban areas; (3) the fact that general hospitals are properly playing an increasing role in the primary care of patients with tuberculosis, and are thus exposing increasing numbers of tuberculin-negative personnel to unsuspected and known tuberculosis patients; and (4) the fact that isoniazid treatment is not without some risk.

The Committee on Infections Within Hospitals of the American Hospital Association, after consultation and consideration of the available data, concluded that BCG vaccination should be considered for use in tuberculin-negative hospital personnel in certain areas. These areas and circumstances are more fully defined in the next section.

WHICH APPROACH SERVES BEST IN A GIVEN LOCALE?

Springett (ref. 25) has critically reviewed the circumstances under which the use of BCG vaccine should be considered. He concluded that in communities or age groups in which annual tuberculin conversion rates are expected to be 0.5 per cent to one per cent or more, BCG vaccination is justified. Where skin-test conversion rates are less than 0.5 per cent, the tuberculosis attack rate in tuberculin-negative individuals becomes so low that BCG vaccination is no longer economically justified. Admittedly, these considerations were applied to communities, but they can be applied with some validity to the "community" of tuberculin-negative hospital personnel.

Hospitals serving communities or populations in which the endemic occurrence of tuberculosis is minimal and in which the skin-test conversion rate among tuberculin-negative employees is less than one per cent per year are well advised to continue a regular program of tuberculin skin testing and isoniazid treatment of converters. Hospitals serving major urban population centers, particularly those with large ghetto, skid row, or derelict, populations, in which the endemic incidence of tuberculosis is relatively high, are urged to consider using BCG vaccine when the skin-test conversion rate among tuberculin-negative employees is demonstrated to exceed one per cent per year.

Of overriding importance in a tuberculosis control program for hospital personnel are the vigor and compulsiveness with which it is carried out and followed up. No tuberculosis control program is 100 per cent effective, but maximum effectiveness of either of the available methods of tuberculosis control can be realized only by participation by all personnel. This responsibility must be accepted by the hospital infection committee.

SUMMARY

Because tuberculosis patients are now admitted to general hospitals, an adequate tuberculosis control program for hospital employees grows increasingly important. There are two approaches to control: (1) a systematic program of skin testing of tuberculin-negative employees, coupled with isoniazid treatment of skin-test converters; and (2) BCG vaccination of tuberculin-negative employees, coupled with annual chest x-rays thereafter. Tuberculin-positive employees should have annual chest x-rays under either plan.

The use of BCG vaccine should be considered in hospitals serving populations with a high endemic incidence of clinical tuberculosis and in which the skin-test conversion rate of tuberculin-negative employees exceeds one per cent annually. Regular skin testing and isoniazid prophylaxis constitute the recommended approach in other situations.

Regardless of whether one or both methods of tuberculosis control is adopted, vigorous and compulsive follow-up is the principal determinant of success.

References

1. Guidelines for the general hospital in the admission and care of tuberculous patients. *Amer. Rev. Resp. Dis.* 99:631, 1969.
2. Stead, W. W., and others. Utilization of general hospitals in the treatment of tuberculosis. *Chest.* 61:405, Apr. 1972.
3. Care of patients with pulmonary tuberculosis in general hospitals. Committee on Infections within Hospitals, American Hospital Association. *Hospitals, J.A.H.A.* 46:66, Jan. 16, 1972.
4. Stead, W. W. Pathogenesis of a first episode of chronic pulmonary tuberculosis in man: Recrudescense of residuals of the primary infection or exogenous reinfection? *Amer. Rev. Resp. Dis.* 95:729, 1967.
5. Stead, W. W., and others. Clinical spectrum of primary tuberculosis in adults. Confusion with reinfection in the pathogenesis of chronic tuberculosis. *Ann. Intern. Med.* 68:731, 1968.

6. Edwards, P. Q. Editorial: Tuberculin negative? *New Engl. J. Med.* 286:373, 1972.
7. Preventive therapy of tuberculous infection. A joint statement of the American Lung Association, American Thoracic Society, and Center for Disease Control. *Amer. Rev. Resp. Dis.* 110:371, 1974.
8. Isoniazid and liver disease. Report of the Ad Hoc Committee on Isoniazid and Liver Disease, Center for Disease Control, DHEW, Mar. 17-18, 1971. *Amer. Rev. Resp. Dis.* 104:454, 1971.
9. Smith, J. P., and Scharer, L. Adverse effects of isoniazid and their significance for chemoprophylaxis. *Amer. Rev. Resp. Dis.* 102:821, 1971.
10. Moulding, T. Chemoprophylaxis of tuberculosis: When is the benefit worth the risk and cost? *Ann. Intern. Med.* 74:761, 1971.
11. Ferebee, S. H. Controlled chemoprophylaxis trials in tuberculosis: A general review. *Adv. Tuberc. Res.* 17:28, 1970.
12. Public Health Service recommendations on the use of BCG vaccination in the United States. *Morbidity and Mortality Weekly Report.* 15:350, 1966.
13. Committee on Therapy, American Thoracic Society. Personnel tuberculosis control program in medical institutions. *Amer. Rev. Resp. Dis.* 104:463, 1971.
14. Oatway, W. H. Jr., and others. BCG vaccination. *Amer. Rev. Resp. Dis.* 96:830, 1967.
15. Smith, D. T. Diagnostic and prognostic significance of the quantitative tuberculin tests: The influence of subclinical infections with atypical mycobacteria. *Ann. Intern. Med.* 67:919, 1967.
16. Smith, D. W. Why not vaccinate against tuberculosis? *Ann. Intern. Med.* 72:419, 1970.
17. Smith, D. T. Isoniazid prophylaxis and BCG vaccination in the control of tuberculosis. *Arch. Environ. Health.* 23:235, 1971.
18. Rosenthal, S. R., and others. BCG vaccination against tuberculosis in Chicago: A 20-year study statistically analyzed. *Pediatrics.* 28:622, 1961.
19. Aronson, J. W., and others. A 20-year appraisal of BCG vaccination on the control of tuberculosis. *Arch. Intern. Med.* 101:881, 1958.
20. Dickie, H. A. Tuberculosis in student nurses and medical students at the University of Wisconsin. *Ann. Intern. Med.* 33:941, 1950.
21. Frimodt-Møller, and others. Observations on protective effect of BCG vaccination in south Indian rural population. *Bull. WHO.* 30:545, 1964.

22. BCG and the Vole Bacillus vaccines in the prevention of tuberculosis in adolescence and early adult life: Third report of the Medical Research Council by its Tuberculosis Vaccines Clinical Trials Committee. *Brit. Med. J.* 5336:973, 1963.
23. Comstock, G. W., and Palmer, C. E. Long-term results of BCG vaccination in the southern United States. *Amer. Rev. Resp. Dis.* 93:171, 1966.
24. Comstock, G. W., and Webster, R. G. Tuberculosis studies in Muscogee County, Georgia: VII. A 20-year evaluation of BCG vaccination in a school population. *Amer. Rev. Resp. Dis.* 100:839, 1969.
25. Springett, V. H. The value of BCG vaccination. *Tubercle.* 46:76, 1965.

Appendix D

GUIDELINES ON HEPATITIS B ANTIGEN CARRIERS

In January 1971 the American Hospital Association sent a *Statement on Screening Donor Blood for Hepatitis B Associated Antigen* (hepatitis B antigen, HB Ag, Australia antigen) to all hospitals. This statement emphasized the magnitude of the problem of hepatitis B associated with blood transfusions; and indicated blood containing it should not be transfused. Subsequently, the use of a test for HB Ag has become recognized as essential in each hospital blood banking service in order to reduce the risk of hepatitis B to patients and personnel. The hepatitis B antigen is an indicator of the presence of the hepatitis B (HBV serum hepatitis) virus. A widely used HB Ag test utilizes counter-immunoelectrophoresis (CEP), but it identifies only 20 per cent to 50 per cent of infected blood. The most sensitive tests include reversed passive hemagglutination (RPHA) or radio-immunoassay (RIA). These identify a greater portion of, but not all, blood infected with HBV.

It should be remembered that hepatitis A (infectious hepatitis) can also be transmitted parenterally. Although it is clear that the major route of transmission of hepatitis A is enteric and that of hepatitis B is parenteral, either can be transmitted by the other route. The current inability to

---

Approved by American Hospital Association General Council, Oct. 25, 1974.

identify hepatitis A in blood may explain a portion of the cases of HB Ag-negative posttransfusion hepatitis.

With donated blood now being tested routinely, and with the frequent use of sensitive HB Ag tests in diagnosis and evaluation of various clinical problems, queries have arisen concerning how to handle a hospital employee or patient without clinical hepatitis who is HB Ag positive. The definitive answers to these queries remain to be developed. At this time the following guidelines have been designed to minimize realistically the risk of hepatitis B being spread.

General Management of Patients or Personnel Who Are Positive for HB Ag

If the individual found positive for HB Ag is asymptomatic, the test should be repeated. If the positive result is confirmed, he should be evaluated for active subclinical liver disease and treated appropriately. If no evidence of liver disease is found, he may be considered a carrier, and is likely to remain a carrier indefinitely. However, he may be recovering from subclinical hepatitis and should be retested for HB Ag three and six months later. Most patients who revert to negative after recovery from hepatitis B do so within three months. Once HB Ag is no longer demonstrable, these individuals are not believed to be dangerous, except possibly as blood donors. *No one who is or is known to have been HB Ag positive should ever donate blood for transfusion.*

There is no evidence that commercial gamma globulin is useful in the management of patients or carriers positive for HB Ag, and it is not recommended for prophylaxis of contacts of these individuals.

Special Management of Hospitalized Patients Who Are Positive for HB Ag

To prevent hepatitis B in hospital employees, measures should be instituted to minimize unnecessary staff contact with positive patients and positive blood. When contact is necessary, specific precautions should be taken to prevent transmission of the virus. Parenteral inoculation of blood or serum is considered the most important but not the only mechanism of spread of hepatitis B. Oral transmission via ingestion of HB Ag-positive material has been demonstrated experimentally. Since inoculation of as little as 0.0001 milliliters of HB Ag-positive serum can transmit the disease, persons handling positive blood specimens in laboratories may acquire the infection via minor cuts and abrasions in skin or mucous membranes or via hand to mouth transfer of small amounts of blood. Occasional transmission of the virus by other nonparenteral means, such as by transfer across mucous membranes or via the airborne route, is also considered possible. No outbreaks of hepatitis B have been reported that have been traced to contaminated food or water. Patients with overt hepatitis or who are bleeding are probably more likely to transmit the disease than healthy carriers. The exact frequency and the overall importance of the various modes of nonparenteral transmission remain undetermined.

Although routine testing of patients and personnel is not recommended at this time, it is recommended that all patients in hospitals who are known to be positive for HB Ag should be handled in a fashion similar to patients with overt hepatitis. Blood precautions and enteric precautions should be used.

Persons working in dialysis units develop HB Ag-positive hepatitis (clinical or subclinical) more frequently than the general population does, partly because dialysis patients frequently carry the antigen and partly because the workers frequently have contact with blood during various dialysis procedures. Persons having frequent or heavy contact with blood or blood products, such as those working in dialysis units and certain laboratories, should wear appropriate protective clothing (gowns, scrub suits, or laboratory coats) and should wear protective gloves. Eating, drinking, and smoking should be prohibited in these and other areas where contact with blood occurs, so as to minimize the transfer of small amounts of blood or serum from hands to mouth. Rubber bulbs should be used for pipetting blood. The importance of careful hand washing after contact with blood should be stressed. Because there are patients who are undetected carriers of HB Ag, *all* blood specimens should be considered potentially infectious (even if tested and found negative for HB Ag). *Although there is no substitute for careful handling of all blood specimens, adequate provision should be made to warn hospital personnel likely to contact patients with positive HB antigenemia or biologic materials derived from such patients.*

Contamination with hepatitis B antigen of laboratory reagents used in testing for hepatitis B antigen or antibody is a special problem. Reports indicate that more than 50 per cent of such reagents are so contaminated. Until further information is available, all such reagents should be handled as if they were contaminated.

Surgeons should be made aware of their special risk of acquiring hepatitis from patients who are HB Ag positive, particularly when wire sutures are used for wound closure, presumably because of the frequency of puncture of gloves and skin while tying wire.

Special Management of HB Ag-Positive Personnel

The hospital employee confirmed as an asymptomatic, or healthy, carrier of HB Ag presents a problem different from that of patients, who can be isolated with relative ease. Presently, the infectious potential of personnel carriers of HB Ag for patients and other contacts is unknown, and we cannot make definitive statements concerning restrictions with regard to their activities. It is clear that direct contact with their blood or serum is hazardous; they should not donate blood. As indicated earlier, nonparenteral transmission of the virus is possible. The epidemiologic evidence suggests positive personnel are less infectious than positive patients. In the reported instances of spread by direct contact, the individual who was the source of HB Ag had acute hepatitis or a hemorrhagic diathesis.

On the basis of presently available data, otherwise healthy carriers should be allowed to work in the hospital without restrictions. They should be advised of the carrier state and told that they should not donate blood. As with all personnel who have patient care responsibilities, they should be advised to practice strict personal hygiene and to exercise care in preventing their blood or secretions from contacting other individuals. Although carriers should be made aware of the potential for problems, they should not be ostracized, but should be followed, reevaluated, and counseled. All HB Ag-positive personnel should be subject to this kind of surveillance.

Because restrictions on personnel who are positive are not advised, a program of routine testing of personnel for HB Ag does not seem necessary at this time. The routine testing of all patients is also not advised. Only about 0.1 per cent to 0.2 per cent of healthy adults or hospitalized patients without liver disease are positive. Periodic testing may be worth while for high-risk groups, such as patients or personnel in dialysis programs, and patients with liver disease of uncertain etiology.

The infection committee should be notified by the laboratory of all positive tests for HB Ag and should initiate a follow-up investigation of these reports as part of its surveillance activity. All cases of hepatitis B should be investigated and potential sources identified. If any cases of hepatitis B are thought to be related to personnel or members of the staff who are HB Ag positive, a careful reassessment should be made. In this unusual circumstance, it may be wise to have the individual reassigned to a function with minimal or no patient contact for as long as the HB Ag carrier state persists. Other, less drastic control measures may also be suitable, depending on the situation.

Appendix E

NOMENCLATURE OF ANTIGENS ASSOCIATED WITH VIRAL HEPATITIS TYPE B

In April 1972, the Committee on Viral Hepatitis of the National Research Council employed in its first publication (ref. 1), the descriptive terms HB Ag and HB Ab for the antigen and antibody associated with viral hepatitis type B. Since then, growing evidence of the complexity of the antigen has highlighted the need to modify this nomenclature. It has been clearly established that the 42-nm structure now known as the Dane particle and the 20-nm spherical and filamentous particles are associated with viral hepatitis type B. The Dane particle consists of a core and an

---

This statement, published in *Morbidity and Mortality Weekly Report* 23:4, Jan. 26, 1974, was made possible by funds provided under a contract with the National Institutes of Health (PH43-64-44, task order 56). It was prepared by the Committee on Viral Hepatitis of the National Research Council—National Academy of Sciences. Committee members were:

Saul Krugman, M.D., chairman, Department of Pediatrics, New York University School of Medicine, New York; Michael B. Gregg, M.D., Center for Disease Control, Atlanta; Elvin A. Kabat, Ph.D., Department of Microbiology, College of Physicians and Surgeons, Columbia University, New York City; Robert W. McCollum, M.D., Department of Epidemiology and Public Health, Yale University School of Medicine, New Haven, Conn.; Joseph L. Melnick, Ph.D., Department of Virology and Epidemiology, Baylor College of Medicine, Houston, Tex.; Allan G. Redeker, M.D., Department of Medicine, University of Southern California, Los Angeles; and Patricia E. Taylor, Ph.D., Laboratory Centre for Disease Control, Ottawa, Ont., Canada.

outer surface component each having specific antigenic properties. The surface component is antigenically similar to the 20-nm particles. The 20-nm particles appear to be formed as the result of overproduction of the surface component of the Dane particle. In addition, it has been established that this surface antigen manifests a group-specific determinant, a, and subtype-specific determinants, d or y, and w or r.

In view of these circumstances and in expectation of continuing revelations in this field, the committee believes that scientific communication would be greatly enhanced by the acceptance of a standard nomenclature adaptable to newly discovered antigens, antibodies, or viruses. We therefore suggest that consideration be given the following system of nomenclature.

HB_s Ag	The hepatitis B antigen found on the surface of the Dane particle and on the unattached 20-nm particles.
HB_c Ag	The hepatitis B antigen found within the core of the Dane particle.
Dane particle	A current term for the 42-nm particle containing HB_c Ag in its core and HB_s Ag on its surface.
HBV	Reserved for hepatitis B virus. The Dane particle may turn out to be HBV.
HB_s Ag/adr	Hepatitis B surface antigen manifesting the group-specific determinant, a, and subtype-specific determinants, d and r. All recognized subtypes are to be indicated to the right of the slash.
anti-HB_s	Antibody to hepatitis B surface antigen. If the subtypic reactivity is known, the appropriate antigenic determinants are to be indicated to the right of a slash.
anti-HB_c	Antibody to hepatitis B core antigen. If more than one core antigen is discovered, the corresponding antigens can be indicated.

The present use of HB Ab in designating the antibody to hepatitis B antigen should be abandoned.

Reference

1. Committee on Viral Hepatitis, National Academy of Sciences. The public health implications of the presence of hepatitis B antigen in human serum. *Morbidity and Mortality Weekly Report* 21:133, 1972.

Glossary

Antiseptic—A chemical compound that stops or inhibits the growth of bacteria without necessarily killing them. The term is usually reserved for compounds applied to living tissue.

Asepsis—The exclusion of microorganisms causing infection.

Attack rate, also see *Incidence* and *Prevalence*—A figure reflecting the number of cases of a particular disease or infection in proportion to the total number of individuals at risk during a specified period. For example:

$$\text{Attack rate} = \frac{\text{Number of new infections}}{\text{Number of patients in hospital}} \times 100 \text{ (expressed as \%)}$$

Carrier—An infected person who harbors a specific infectious agent without having a discernible clinical disease and serves as a potential source of infection for others. Carriers with inapparent infections are commonly known as healthy carriers. Carriers in the incubatory or convalescent stage of a clinically recognizable disease are known as incubatory and convalescent carriers. Under either circumstance the carrier state may be of short or long duration, as in the case of temporary or chronic carriers. Vertebrate animals other than man may also be carriers.

Commensal—An organism living on and/or within another and deriving benefit from the host but not causing injury to it.

Communicable disease—An illness that is due to a specific infectious agent or its toxic products and that results from transmission of that agent or its products from a reservoir to a susceptible host, either directly, as from an infected person or animal, or indirectly, through the agency of an intermediate plant or animal host, a vector, or the inanimate environment.

Compromised host—A person whose defense mechanism against disease is deficient.

Contact—A person or animal in such association with an infected person or animal or a contaminated environment as to have opportunity to acquire infection. Direct exposure may involve physical contact. Indirect exposure, with no established physical touching, comes through living in the same household or being in the same room or associating at school, work, or play. Exposure may be long or short; single, continued, or repetitive; and casual or close. To express degrees of risk of developing infection, such indirectly exposed persons are often denoted either as familial, school, or work contacts or as close, casual, or remote contacts.

Contagious—Applies to a disease that is communicable or capable of being transmitted from one person or animal to another person or animal.

Contamination—The presence of an infectious agent on a body surface; also on or in clothes, bedding, toys, surgical instruments, or dressings, or on or in other inanimate articles or substances, including air, water, milk, and food. Contamination is distinct from pollution, which implies the presence of offensive but noninfectious matter in the environment.

Detergent—A water soluble or liquid organic surface-active agent for washing. It resembles soap in its ability to emulsify oils and hold dirt in suspension, but does not precipitate calcium and magnesium salts.

Disinfectant—A chemical substance that inhibits or destroys microorganisms. The term is usually reserved for substances suitable for application to inanimate objects.

Disinfection—The killing of infectious agents outside the body by chemical or physical means directly applied.

Ecology—A branch of science concerned with the interrelationship of organisms and their environment.

Endemic—The habitual presence of a disease within a geographic area; may also refer to the usual prevalence of a given disease within such an area.

Endogenous infection—An infection resulting from bacteria normally resident in the host.

Epidemic—An outbreak in a community or region of a group of illnesses of similar nature, clearly in excess of normal expectancy and derived from a common or a propagated source.

Epidemiology—The study of occurrence and distribution of disease.

Exogenous infection—An infection resulting from contamination by a source outside the patient.

Fomites (singular: fomes)—Any article or substance other than food that may transmit infectious organisms.

Germicide—An agent that destroys germs.

Inapparent infection—The presence of infection in a host without occurrence of recognizable clinical signs or symptoms. Inapparent infections are specifically identifiable by laboratory means.

Incidence—A general term for the frequency of occurrence of a disease, infection, or other event over a period of time and in relation to the population in which it occurs. Incidence is expressed more specifically as a rate, commonly the number of new cases during a prescribed time for a specific unit of population. An example is cases of tuberculosis per 100,000 population per year.

Infection—The entry and development or multiplication of an infectious agent in the body of a person or an animal. Infection is not synonymous with infectious disease; the result of infection may be inapparent or manifest. The presence of living infectious agents on exterior surfaces of the body or on articles of apparel or on soiled articles is not infection, but contamination. The term *infection* should not be used to describe conditions of inanimate matter such as soil, water, sewage, milk, or food; the term *contamination* applies.

Isolation—The separation of infected persons from other persons in such places and under such conditions as will prevent direct or indirect conveyance of the infectious agent from infected persons to persons who are susceptible or who may spread the agent to others. The duration of isolation is usually for the period of communicability.

Microbial load—The number of microorganisms with which an object is contaminated.

Nosocomial—Arising within a hospital.

Prevalence—A general term to characterize the frequency of a disease or other event at a particular time and in relation to a particular population. Prevalence is expressed more specifically as a ratio; a prevalence ratio is the number of cases of disease present in a specified population at a particular time.

Protoplast—An atypical osmotically fragile bacterium lacking a cell wall; sometimes called L form.

RODAC plate—A special dish used for culturing the environment and in which the agar extends above the edge of the dish. (RODAC stands for replicate organism detection and counting.)

Saprophyte—Any vegetable organism, such as a bacterium, living upon dead or decaying organic matter.

Sterile—Free from microorganisms.

Sterilization—The rendering of an object or material free from living organisms.

Surveillance of disease—The continuing scrutiny of all aspects of occurrence and spread of disease that are pertinent to effective control. Included are the systematic collection and evaluation of morbidity and mortality reports; of special reports of field investigations, epidemics, and individual cases; of reports of isolations and identifications of infectious agents in laboratories; of data concerning the availability and use of vaccines, immune globulin, insecticides, and other substances used in control; of information regarding immunity levels in segments of the population; and of other relevant epidemiologic data. A regular summary report of these data should be prepared and distributed to appropriate individuals.

Index

Active immunization, of personnel, 29-30
Administrative nurse, responsibilities of, 43
Airborne contamination, 78-79
  sources and control (table), 78
Anesthesia
  care of equipment, 143-44
  as hazardous procedure, 141-44
  special procedures for, 142-43
Antibiotic prophylaxis, 91-93
Antibiotics
  as therapeutic procedure, 9
  monitored usage of, 20
  and resistant microorganisms, 91
Antimicrobial agents
  given prophylactically, 15
  resistance to, 6
Antimicrobial chemicals, evaluation of (table), 106-07
Antimicrobial drugs
  dispensed by the pharmacy, 49
  effectiveness of, 91
Antisepsis, 107-11
Antiseptics
  as bacteriostatic agents, 108-09
  in vitro trials of, 47
Architectural and design considerations, 69-77
Asepsis, in surgical suite, 127-29
Autoclaves, 96

Bacterial endocarditis, preventive measures for, 91
Bleaches, in decontamination, 110
Blood bank, as hazardous area, 124-26
Blood donors, rejection of, 125-26
Building design
  floor plan for isolation room (fig.), 77
  in infection control, aspects of, 76-77
Burn treatment areas, related to visitors, 36

Carpets, advantages and disadvantages of, 75-76
Carriers of infection, 119-24
  asymptomatic, 119-20
  management of personnel, 123-24

routine search for, 120
specific search for, 120-23
Catheterization, as hazardous procedure, 149
Central supply service, responsibilities of, 50-52
Chemical disinfectants
  effect of temperature on, 104
  neutralization of, 104, 107
Chlorine, as decontaminating agent, 110
Clean linen, storage of, 58-59
Cohort plan, in nursery management, 136
Committee on Infections Within Hospitals (AHA), 19
Compromised host
  defined, 12
  factors predisposing to infection (table), 11
Conveyors and dumbwaiters, as design factors, 70-71

Daily work sheet, as record of infection, 21, 22 (fig.), 23
Darling v. Charleston Community Memorial Hospital, 18 n.
Diagnostic procedures, as hazards, 9
Dialysis unit
  as hazardous area, 133-35
  precautions in, 184
Disinfectants
  in contaminated areas, 61
  in vitro trials of, 47
Disinfection, 93-94, 102-05
  by chemical agents, 103-04
  of instruments (table), 108-09
  by physical agents, 102-03

Employees. *See also* Personnel
  with communicable diseases, 56
  education programs for, 31-34
  health service for, 27-31
  tuberculosis control programs for, 171-79
Engineering and maintenance, departmental responsibilities of, 63-64

Environmental control, 78-80
Environmental sanitation. *See* Housekeeping
Epidemiologist
  in infection control, 20
  responsibilities of, 41-42
Epidemiology of infection. *See* Nosocomial infection, epidemiologic problems of
Equipment and instruments, in the surgical suite, 129-31
Equipment and supplies, in the isolation room, 87

Finish materials, as design factors, 74-75
Fogging. *See* Housekeeping, fogging
Fomites, defined, 6
Food service
  departmental responsibilities, 52-56
  equipment for, 54
  preparation of food, 55
  principles of protection, 53-54
  responsibilities of director, 56
  serving food, 55-56
  storage, 55

Gastroenteritis, precautions for, 82
Gonorrhea, prophylactic treatment for, 91-92

Hand washing, 111-13
  aids, 111-12
  facilities, 76
  techniques, 112-13
Hazardous areas, 124-41
Hazardous procedures, 141-54
Hepatitis, 7, 28, 30, 82, 133-34
  infectious, 182
  nomenclature for antigens, 186-87
  patient carriers, 183-84
  personnel carriers, 184-85
  posttransfusion, 125
  in search for carriers, 123
  statement on carriers, 182-85
  testing for, 182-85
  viral, 82 (fig.), 186-87

Hexachlorophene
  as antiseptic, 110
  in infant's bath, 139
Hospital-acquired infection. *See* Nosocomial infection
Hospital administrator, responsibilities of, 39-40
Hospital employees. *See* Employees; Personnel
Hospital staff. *See* Employees; Personnel
Hospitals
  medicolegal responsibilities of, 17-19
  responsibilities within, 39-64
  standards for care, 17-19
Hospitals, J.A.H.A., recommendations on infection control, 19
Housekeeping
  cleaning agents and apparatus, 61
  cleaning routines, 59-60
  departmental responsibilities, 59-63
  fogging, 60, 62-63
  general rules, 60-61
Hyperalimentation. *See* Total parenteral nutrition

Immunosuppressive drugs, 9
Infants
  as carriers, 140-41
  protection of, 135
Infected patient. *See also* Carriers of infection
  in operating room, 131
Infected personnel. *See* Carriers of infection
Infection. *See also* Nosocomial infection
  by airborne organisms, 8
  appearing after hospitalization, 6
  appearing during hospitalization, 5
  common vehicle for, defined, 8
  by direct contact, 7
  droplet-spread, 7-8
  environment as factor in, 9
  epidemiology of, 5-15
  factors influencing, 6-9
  host susceptibility, 9
  incidence of, 119
  indirect spread of, 7
  model for transmission of (fig.), 32
  organisms frequently implicated in (table), 13
  predisposing factors related to microorganisms 14 (table), 15
  present on admission, 5
  related to isolation, 81
  related to therapeutic measures (table), 12
  route of transmission, 7-9
  sources of, 6
  susceptibility to, 2
  transmission patterns, 31-32
  types of, 5
  vectorborne, 8
Infection control committee
  guidelines for, 19-20
  and nursery infections, 141
  responsibilities of, 19-20
  in search for carriers, 120-23
  supervision of tuberculosis patients, 162
  and testing for hepatitis, 185
Infection control, epidemiologic principles, 10
Infection control nurse
  assisting infection control committee, 20
  in infection control, 20
  participant in training, 33-34
  responsibilities of, 23-27, 44-45
Infectious hepatitis. *See* Hepatitis
Infectious organisms
  commensals, 12
  pseudomonas, 15
  salmonella, 6, 122, 124
  saprophytes, 12
  shigella, 6, 122, 124
  staphylococci, 6, 7, 9, 47, 61, 78, 111, 119, 120-22, 124, 128, 148
  streptococci, 61, 78, 101, 119, 122, 148, 152
  tubercle bacilli, 78
Informal monitoring, of employees, 34
Inhalation therapy
  equipment, 15
  as hazardous procedure, 144-46

Insect control. *See* Vermin, control of
Inservice training programs, for personnel, 33-34
Instruments, chemical disinfection and sterilization (table), 108-09
Intensive care unit
  as hazardous area, 131-33
  and isolation, 90
Intestinal tract, in search for carriers, 122-23
Ionizing radiation. *See* Sterilization, radiation
Isolation
  cost of, 90
  enteric precautions (fig.), 82
  equipment and supplies for, 87
  in intensive care units, 90
  ordered by attending physician, 81
  procedures posted, 87
  protective measures, 81, 82-86 (fig.), 87
  respiratory, 84 (fig.), 87
  reverse, 83 (fig.), 88-89
  role of infection control committee, 80-81
  simplified procedures for, 89-90
  specific precautions, 87
  strict, 85 (fig.), 87
  techniques and procedures, 80-90
  and visitors, 88
  wound and skin precautions (fig.), 86
Isolation unit
  for infant care, 137
  related to visitors, 36

Joint Commission on Accreditation of Hospitals (JCAH), on hospital responsibilities, 17-19

Laundering procedures, 57-58
Laundry and linen service, responsibilities of, 56-59
Laundry and trash chutes, as design factors, 70-71

Malaria, as vectorborne disease, 8
Materials handling, as design factor, 70-71

Medical examinations, of prospective employees, 27-28
Meningococcal infection, prophylaxis for, 92
Microbial agents, as factors influencing infection, 6-7
Microbiological laboratory
  implementing safety measures in, 48-49
  responsibilities of, 46-49
Microbiological sampling, 167-70
Microorganisms
  antibiotic-resistant strains, 9
  as pathogens, 10, 12

Nebulizers
  gas-driven, 146
  ultrasonic, 15, 146
Nonsterile materials, handling of, 51
Nosocomial infection
  cost of, 2-3
  defined, 5
  effectiveness of control program, 157-59
  epidemiologic problems of, 5-15
  incidence of, 2
  motivational influences on control, 158
  reporting of, 17-27
Nursery, newborn
  design, related to infection control, 135-36
  as hazardous area, 135-41
  for high-risk infants, 137-38
  observation, 138
  personnel, health records of, 6
  problems of infection, 140-41
  procedures for, 138-39
  related to visitors, 36
  special units in, 136-38
  suspect, 137
Nursing staff, responsibilities of, 42-46

Operating room
  clothing for, 142
  related to visitors, 36
Opportunistic infections
  defined, 12
  reduction of, 15

Opportunistic pathogens, organisms frequently implicated (table), 13
Orientation program, for new personnel, 33

Passive immunization, of personnel, 30
Pediatrics department, related to visiting privileges, 36
Personnel. *See also* Employees
  carriers of hepatitis, 184-85
  carriers of infection, 119-24
  immunization of, 29-30
  medical treatment of, 28
  monitoring of, 31
  practices in surgical suite, 129
Pharmacy, responsibilities of, 49-50
Physicians, responsibilities of, 40-41
Pneumonia
  and anesthetics, 15
  and isolation, 81
Postoperative wound infection, prophylaxis for, 92-93
Practicing nurse, responsibilities of, 43-44
Prepackaged materials, handling of, 51
Presterilized materials, handling of, 51-52
Procedure manuals, for personnel, 33
Procedures and Layout for the Infant Formula Room (AHA), 139
Protective isolation
  procedures for, 89
  purpose of, 88
Public health nurse, responsibilities of, 45-46

Recovery rooms, related to visitors, 36
Reporting of infection, 21, 22 (fig.), 23, 24-25 (fig.)
Respiratory tract, examined for carrier states, 120-22
Reverse isolation. *See* Protective isolation
Rodent control. *See* Vermin, control of

Salmonella derby, epidemic of, 9
Salmonellosis
  and isolation, 81
  in personnel, 28

Sanitation, in isolation room, 87-88
Scouring powders, in decontamination, 110
Septicemia
  and total parenteral nutrition, 153
  transmission of, 7
Service-pathogen grid chart, in analysis of infection frequency, 23
Shigellosis
  and isolation, 81
  transmission of, 8
Smallpox
  and isolation, 81
  vaccine procedure, 30
Soiled linens, handling of, 56-57
Special-care areas, related to visitors, 36
Spores, survival of, 98
Standards for infection control
  by Joint Commission on Accreditation of Hospitals, 17-20
  under state licensing regulations, 17-19
Staphylococcal gastroenteritis, transmission of, 8
Staphylococcal sepsis
  apparent after discharge, 6
  related to catheters, 152
Staphylococcus aureus, and possible epidemic, 10
Static electricity, in carpets, 76
Sterile supplies, handling of, 52
Sterilization
  background and definition, 93-94
  efficiency of, 47
  ethylene oxide, 98-100
  failure of, 97-98
  high-vacuum, 96-97
  of instruments (table), 108-09
  levels, 94
  radiation, 100-02
  steam, 95-96
  techniques for, 95-102
  ultraviolet radiation, 103
Streptococcal infection, prophylaxis for, 92

Index / 197

Surface contamination, control of, 79-80
Surgical dressing
  as hazardous procedure, 148-49
  techniques for (table), 149
Surgical suite, as hazardous area, 126-31
Surveillance programs, in infection control, 21-23
Syphilis, tests and treatment for, 93

Team Up to Control Infection (Hospital Research and Educational Trust), 34
Therapeutic measures, as factors predisposing to infection (table), 12
Total parenteral nutrition
  defined, 153
  as source of infection, 153-54
TPN. *See* Total parenteral nutrition
Tracheostomy, as hazardous procedure, 146-48
Traffic patterns, of persons, 69-70
Tuberculosis
  BCG (Bacille Calmette-Guerin) vaccine, 29, 174-75, 177-79
  care of patients, 161-66
  control programs for employees, 177-79
  evaluation and follow-up, 93
  hospital measures, 163-65
  inhospital services for, 162-63
  isoniazid prophylaxis, 173, 175-76, 178-79
  reporting and posthospital care, 165-66
  risk among personnel, 172-73
  surveillance and control, 173-75
  surveillance of staff, 165
  tuberculin skin testing, 27, 173-74

Unidirectional (laminar) clean airflow, purpose of, 73-74
Urinary catheters, guidelines for, 149-51

Venous catheters, guidelines for, 151-53
Ventilation systems, as microbial contamination factor, 71-72, 136
Vents and filters, as factors in contamination, 71-72
Vermin, control of, 80
Viral hepatitis. *See* Hepatitis
Visiting hours, 35
Visitors
  as carriers of infection, 119
  in isolation rooms, 88
  policies for, 35
  regulations for, 34-36

Weakened patient. *See* Compromised host

Zoning, of air systems, 72